A YOUNG MAN'S
GUIDE TO SEX

A YOUNG MAN'S GUIDE TO SEX

JAY GALE, PH.D.

The Body Press
Price Stern Sloan
Los Angeles

Published by
THE BODY PRESS
A division of Price Stern Sloan, Inc.
360 North La Cienega Boulevard
Los Angeles, California 90048

Reprinted by arrangement with Henry Holt and Company, Inc.

Library of Congress Cataloging-in-Publication Data

Gale, Jay.
    A young man's guide to sex / Jay Gale.
    p.   cm.
    Reprint. Originally published: New York, Holt, Rinehart, and Winston c1984.
    Bibliography: p.
    Includes index.
    Summary: A comprehensive guide to sex and sexuality, especially for young men, with discussions of sexual truths and lies, masturbation, AIDS, pregnancy, abortion, heterosexuality and homosexuality, and the importance of open communication.
    ISBN 0-89586-691-9: $7.95 ($10.95 Can.)
    1. Sex instruction for boys. 2. Young men—Sexual behavior—Juvenile literature. 3. AIDS (Disease)—Prevention—Juvenile literature.   [1. Sex instruction for boys.]   I. Title.
HQ41.G35 1988
613.9'53—dc19   87-29905
                                                                          CIP
                                                                          AC

Illustrations by Scott E. Carroll
Printed in U.S.A.
1st Printing
10 9 8 7 6 5 4 3 2 1

Grateful acknowledgment is made to the
following for permission to reprint excerpts
from their publications:
Centers for Disease Control: Division of
Venereal Disease Control, for graphs based on
information in STD Statistical Letter C.Y. 1982.
Kinsey Institute for Research in Sex, Gender
& Reproduction, Inc., for graph
adapted from *Sexual Behavior in the Human Male*,
by A. C. Kinsey et al., W. B. Saunders, 1948.
Alfred A. Knopf, Inc., for excerpt from *The Hite Report
on Male Sexuality*, by Shere Hite, Copyright © 1978,
1981 by Shere Hite.
Julius Lester, for excerpt from "Being a Boy,"
which appeared in *Ms.*, July 1973.
Little, Brown and Company, for excerpt from
Male Sexuality, by Bernie Zilbergeld,
Copyright © 1978 by Bernie Zilbergeld.
Macmillan Publishing Co., Inc., for excerpt from
Teenage Sexuality, by Aaron Hass, Ph.D.,
Copyright © 1979 by Aaron Hass, Ph.D.
SAH Enterprises, Inc., for excerpt from
"The Regular Way," by Bill Cosby, which appeared
in *Playboy*, December 1968.
Simon and Schuster, for excerpt from *Fast Times
at Ridgemont High*, by Cameron Crowe,
Copyright © 1981 by Cameron Crowe.

To Fran,
who taught me all about loving,
and to Scott and Erica,
who helped me learn
how to share it

CONTENTS

Contents

ILLUSTRATIONS

ACKNOWLEDGMENTS

The knowledge and wisdom of hundreds of professionals, accumulated over a number of years, and the support of many friends have made this book a published reality. When it comes time to acknowledge them, a few people stand out.

To the members of La Paz Psychological Group in Mission Viejo, California—Robert Solnick, Ph.D.; Jerry Smith, M.A.; Sheila Church, M.A.; and Nancy Recht, M.A.—and to Robert Olson, Ph.D., a special thanks for their professional expertise and evaluation of the manuscript and for their unflagging emotional support.

Also, to Sandra Watt, my eternal gratefulness for her confidence and persistence, which enabled this book to become more than my own private treatise.

Finally, to Tracy Bernstein, Jacque Voss, and especially Bobbi Mark for incredible patience, invaluable professional expertise, and friendship through some very difficult periods.

A YOUNG MAN'S
GUIDE TO SEX

INTRODUCTION

Learning about sex is awfully confusing. All around you are movies, magazines, and advertisements telling how sex is fun and exciting. Yet, as soon as you want to find out what it is all about, adults start talking about marriage, morals, pregnancy, and venereal disease and make sex seem dull or dangerous. This book, however, confirms what your mind has been telling you all along. Sex *can* be fun and exciting.

It is realistic to say that whether through intercourse, masturbation, or plain old "making out," virtually every boy will engage in some sexual activity before marriage. Sex is not something that occurs only after marriage for the purpose of having babies. This is a book about your sexuality and is *not* a book about marriage or pregnancy. It also doesn't try to teach how you *ought* to behave sexually, though it does point out some important responsibilities that go along with sex. Basically, it is designed to help you find your own values.

In presenting my own ideas about sex, I in no way

want to indicate that my way of looking at sex is the only way or even the right way. In this book I present what many or most teenagers experience, but you are a unique individual. Consequently, your experiences will differ to some degree from those of other adolescents. I hope that after reading this book you will find that you are the only true expert on your body and feelings.

There are two levels of information required to understand your sexual self. One is the "mechanical information" that enables you to find out what to do. This is the level where you learn, for instance, how to make love or how babies are conceived. The other is the "emotional" information that helps you learn to understand your feelings and conflicts and to begin to put these into perspective.

Understanding the mechanical without the emotional is like having a friend describe the action at an overtime football game. He can explain what happened, but it is nothing like being at the stadium and experiencing the excitement of the competition and the crowd. Understanding the emotional part without having a knowledge of the mechanics is impossible.

Since boys and girls are so different emotionally as well as physically, it is impractical to relate to both in one book. Consequently, unlike most books about sex that are written for both boys and girls, this book is written for and about boys only. It is designed to cover the mechanics of sex, but in addition there are questions, exercises, and text to help you understand what you are going through emotionally.

In reading a book like this one, you may have a tendency to want to look ahead to the "good parts," where I discuss more about the mechanics of making love, or to a chapter that discusses some problem you are presently experiencing. If you need to do that, fine, but don't forget to come back to the chapters you skipped. It is important for you to have a thorough understanding of what you have experienced and are presently experiencing if you are to meet your sexual future with a minimum of hang-ups. The order of these chapters was based on the way I felt they could be most beneficial to you. Again, you are a unique person with unique needs. Consequently, if you do have a different order in mind, please mark each chapter as you read it, so you don't forget to return to the ones you passed by.

Especially important is the final chapter of the book, A New Era In Sexuality: AIDS, Sexual Responsibility, and Safe Sex. Its place at the end of the book in no way indicates a lack of importance. Rather it was placed there to allow the rapidly changing information about AIDS to be updated more easily in future editions of this book. It is essential that you understand this information about AIDS, sexual responsibility, and safer sex precautions before you are ever sexually intimate. Your life may depend on it.

This book provides an opportunity for you to become aware of what you are sexually and to understand what you have been going through. This is not a book that you can read just once and expect to understand everything there is to know about sex. I hope that reading through it a single time will help you clear up much of the confusion that most adolescents experience about sex. To take full advantage of this book, read through the entire book once from cover to cover to become familiar with the information it contains. Then put it away until you enter a different stage of your sexuality. When you feel you are ready, go back and read the chapters that are about the stage you are going through. For instance, if you are just getting into making out, it may be difficult for you to understand the concerns of a teenage boy going through a relationship that involves intercourse with a girl. Wait until you feel you are ready for that chapter, and then go back and read it again.

Because most maturing young males gear their primary sexual interest toward females, references to sexual partners used throughout this text consistently refer to "she," "her," or other feminine pronouns. For those readers whose primary interest is homosexual (sexual interest toward other males) or for some of those who are confused about their sexual preference, substituting masculine pronouns such as "he" or "his" may make it easier to relate to the information in this book.

Each chapter will open new alternatives that you might want to explore and give you a more educated way of choosing the direction you will be taking in the future. As a sexual being you will be growing and changing every day for the rest of your life. You will have failures and successes, and this book can help you learn from both.

1

LEARNING AND COMMUNICATION

Learning about Sex

When I was growing up, I kept thinking that somehow I was going to learn about sex. My parents never mentioned it and I had no books to learn from, but somehow I thought that magically, as I got older, I would understand the strange things that were happening to my mind and body.

None of my teachers ever spoke of sex. Even in the one sex education class I had, sex was not taught. The teacher talked about the reproductive organs of the body as if he were teaching a class in automotive mechanics. I learned where the parts of the body were and how sperm would squiggle their way to the egg to produce an embryo. I learned a little about marriage and the stages of birth, but my sex education was still without any education about sex.

I heard sex joked about and whispered about. My friends lied through their teeth about the size of their penises or how far they could "come." Not only was I impressed, but I was worried. I guessed that they were probably lying, but I wasn't sure. I had no information with which to compare their claims, except for my own body, and I knew that there was no way I could compete. The lies and the facts blended, and what I was left with was confusion.

Unfortunately, my body and my mind couldn't wait to sort the information. My body was changing and my mind was leading me through all sorts of imaginary sexual adventures. I was feeling crazy, driven by all sorts of urges and feelings. I don't think I ever felt so alone. Feeling crazy and confused, I was sure that I was the only person who ever went through such an experience. I needed information, but I had no idea where to get it.

Sharing with Friends

Talking about sex with other boys is a real art. It is difficult to sit around with a group of guys without letting them know how much you don't understand. Some guys will brag about sex, some joke about it, and others simply nod quietly in agreement with everything that is said. They all just sit around acting like they know everything there is to know about sex. Although most boys appear open and comfortable talking and joking about it in a conversation, they tend to be much more secretive than girls. Rarely do boys share their confusion or concerns, especially in a group. In the following article written for *Playboy* magazine in 1968, comedian Bill Cosby shares an experience illustrating this fine art of bluffing.[1]

Rufus ... says, You're goin' with Rosemary, huh? I say, Yeah. He says, Did you get any yet? I say, Get any what? He says, You know, man. I say, No man. I didn't get any ... get any *what?* He says, Did you get any ... p-u-s-s-y. I say, No man I don't do that kind of thing. ...

Now the truth is, I don't know nothin' about p-u-s-s-y. You walk around the neighborhood, you see signs on the sidewalk, on the walls: *Pussy is good.* And it's somethin' that you just take for granted— you look at it and say, Yeah. But most of the kids who write it never had any.

After making arrangements with a girl to "get some p-u-s-s-y" on Saturday, Cosby tries desperately to get information without admitting to anyone that he doesn't have the slightest idea what he is doing.

So Saturday comes and I've been thinking all week about this p-u-s-s-y. You know, and I'm trying to ask people questions about how they get some p-u-s-s-y. And I don't want guys to know that I don't know nothin' about gettin' no p-u-s-s-y. But how do you find out how to do it without blowin' the fact that you don't know how to do it? So I come to a guy and I say, Say man, have you ever had any p-u-s-s-y? And the guy says, Yeah. And I say, Well, man, what's your favorite way of gettin' it? He says, Well, you know, just the regular way. And I say, Well, do you do it like I do it? And the cat says, How's that? And I say, Well hey, I heard that there was different ways of doin' it, man. He says, Well, there's a lotta ways of doin' it, you know, but I think that ... you know, the *regular* way . . . I say *Yeah*, good ol' regular way of gettin' p-u-s-s-y.

Sharing with your friends about sex will be difficult at best. It will take a great deal of trust to admit to being sexually inexperienced or to talk about a lack of understanding about some aspect of sex. Therefore, if you do decide to share your questions and concerns, it is important to choose a friend whom you trust and who you feel will be able to share honestly his own feelings. In addition, since boys tend to talk less openly in a group, speak to your friend in a setting in which the two of you can have an intimate discussion without facing the pressure of insensitive peers.

Even in talking with your friends, however, it is important to take into consideration that your experiences and feelings will not be identical to theirs. Each of you gets turned on or off by different things. A girl that you find attractive may not appeal at all to your friends. Share your feelings with them and listen to what they have to say, but do not judge either them or yourself. Each of you will have different values, different standards, and vastly different backgrounds. Sexually, there is no right or wrong way to believe.

Another aspect of the bragging that boys often engage in is that it creates a great deal of pressure. I remember sitting around "shooting the bull" (and that's exactly what it was) with a bunch of guys, feeling the discomfort of having to lie in order to save face, and experiencing additional pressures from the feelings of inadequacy their stories raised in me. I prayed I would find a nymphomaniac who would teach me everything she knew so that I could catch up with the other guys, but I never found her.

Again, Cosby's writing captures that feeling so well. Reacting to pressure from his friends, Cosby approaches his girlfriend's house.

So I keep walkin', and the closer I get to the house, the more scared I get. And I get to the house, and now *I don't want to do it*. I mean, *I don't want none* 'cause it's nasty . . . and it's *dirty* . . . and you will *go to hell*, and she could get pregnant; and my mother's gonna cry, and my father's gonna cry, and I'll probably get a beatin' . . . so I really don't know what to do now.

In an open and honest discussion, friends can be potentially some of your best resources for checking out your sexual feelings, because they are more than likely going through similar kinds of experiences and emotions as you are. It is more realistic to note, however, that few teenage boys talk openly about sex, and their bragging and exaggerations become more of a source of confusion than of help.

When Will My Parents Teach Me about Sex?

Actually, your parents have been teaching you about sex from the day you were born. The name they chose for you, the blue blanket they wrapped you in, the toys they bought for you, all came with certain expectations of you as a male. It is impossible not to have expectations for a child.

As they are growing up, boys are often raised to be

tough and aggressive and taught that crying and emotionalism are undesirable. Tenderness is rarely as acceptable from a boy as from a girl. Boys have to be "macho." Certainly this can be confusing for a teenager who is beginning to feel tender emotions toward a girl yet won't give himself permission to talk about them for fear of being perceived as unmasculine.

Parents also communicate an acceptance or rejection of a child by the way they hold him and touch him. A mother who feeds her child without holding him or omits numerous feedings may well communicate a rejection to the child, which in later years may affect his self-image.

In addition, parents also model a relationship against which the child will later compare future relationships of his own. If your parents are affectionate and loving, certainly it will make it easier for you to communicate these feelings, because they have been modeled for you. It is like watching a movie character that you really enjoy. By watching him in the movie, you can copy some of the actions and mannerisms you admire. If your parents are comfortable in touching each other and you, then you will probably feel less awkwardness communicating affection through holding and touching.

Talking with Parents about Sex

I have been a sex therapist for about 16 years and consequently have talked to hundreds of people about the most intimate parts of their sexual lives. I have done this so many times that talking about sex is fairly easy for me. But when it comes to my own children, I feel much more discomfort. I am not sure where this uneasiness comes from. I want my children to understand their own sexuality and I want them to feel comfortable with it. Most of all, I want them to be able to share freely with me their questions and experiences. But talking about sex with them still feels difficult.

This discomfort is certainly not universal among parents, but I would guess that most mothers and fathers fall into this category. Often parents awkwardly await the first question about sex from their child, as they look forward to the closeness such intimate discussions bring. Yet, if the question does not come, there is a sense of relief that they did not have to face openly discussing sex.

Even in situations where teenagers do try to discuss sex, the results are not always encouraging. In a survey of teens, Aaron Hass, author of *Teenage Sexuality*, asked the following question: "Have you ever tried to talk openly with either of your parents about sex? If you have tried, how did they respond?" According to Hass, "Forty percent of the boys and 54% of the girls reported attempts to talk openly with a parent. The common parental responses reported by teenagers were the teasing, denial, and the punishment . . . Frequently, a teenager felt lectured instead of listened to."[2]

Let me pose two questions to you.

1. True or false, I would like to be more open with my parents about sex?
2. What have you done to approach your parents about this?

If the answer to question one indicates that you are interested in learning from your parents, then the answer to question two is critical. Many teenagers assume that it is their parents' responsibility to initiate a talk about sex and therefore do nothing about it themselves. If you wish to discuss your questions and concerns about sex, then *you* may have to take the initiative.

Understanding Parents and Siblings

If you have tried in the past to speak with your parents about sex and have not been successful, you and your parents deserve a second chance. If they tease you or make jokes, try to understand that they too may be uncomfortable. Let them know that you are serious. If they present you with a lecture about what is right and wrong, accept this as *their* values. There is no need to convince them that their values are wrong or old-fashioned. You can and will have a different set of values from your parents. That does not mean that one of you is wrong and the other is right. Listen to their values and try to understand what they believe without passing judgment.

Once you understand their values you can evaluate the following:

1. In what areas do my values differ from my parents'?
2. What are the advantages and disadvantages of each of our points of view?

It is important for you to have someone to help you understand what your body and mind are going through. If you choose not to share your questions, concerns, and feelings with your parents or to share only a portion of these with them, then a brother or sister, a friend, a relative, or even a teacher may be a possible alternative.

As with friends, older brothers and sisters can be a valuable source of sexual information, since they may have gone through experiences similar to yours. However, the same cautions that were mentioned about friends apply to brothers and sisters. Realize that both their own comfort or lack of comfort with sex and the circumstances under which you speak to them may affect their honesty and directness in discussing sex with you.

Communicating about Sex

When you send any communication, much more is transmitted than just the words. The tone of your voice, your facial expression, a gesture, a touch, or even the position of your body can change the meaning of a verbal message.

In addition, such reactions as silence, whispering, lying, and joking each serve to communicate a certain discomfort with sex. When your parents are silent about sex, what probably gets communicated is "I am embarrassed about this, and I don't want to talk about it." When your teacher talks about reproduction and marriage rather than sex, the message is "This is related to marriage or having babies. Forget about it for ten years." When your friends lie about their sexual accomplishments, they are saying, "This is an area I feel very uncomfortable and insecure about." In each case what is communicated is very different from what has been said.

Similarly, when you say nothing to your parents, a message also comes through. It may be "I am not interested in sex" or "I know all I need to know about sex," but even in complete silence there *is* communication. There is no such thing as *not* communicating!

Because you *do* communicate with your family and friends about sex in one way or another, you might as well do a good job of it. The following list can be useful in evaluating how well you are communicating about sex. You can either copy the list onto a separate piece of paper or simply do this exercise in your head.

1. In the first column (under the heading "Friends" or "Others") fill in the name of a couple of friends or relatives you feel close to.

2. In the next column, "Message Communicated," write what you feel your words and actions communicate to that person about your interests and attitudes about sex.

3. In a third column, "Intended Communication," write what you feel that you would *like* to communicate to each of these people about your interests and attitudes about sex.

If your responses in columns two and three are consistent, then you are communicating accurately. If, on the other hand, there is a gap between what you are communicating and what you would like to communicate, then the following list of suggestions may be helpful to you in opening up some doors to communicating about sex.

Suggestions and Guidelines

1. Make a list of the areas of sexuality that are most confusing to you, writing down the areas of concern or questions that occur to you.

2. For each item on your list, write down who you feel would have the most information about that topic.

3. Evaluate whether you feel that person would be willing to exchange thoughts, information, and ideas with you. If not, cross that name off and write down another one.

4. For each area of concern or question on your list, evaluate whether you prefer to approach that person whose name you wrote down or whether the risk is too great.

5. If you choose to approach, pick a time and place where the two of you can have a comfortable discussion without being interrupted or feeling rushed.

6. Make a clear statement to that person of what you want to know or want to share.

7. It is hoped that you will get the information you wish. However, be aware that the person you choose may not have the information you wish or you may find their values to be very different from yours.

8. No matter what they say, *listen* without trying to establish a "right" or "wrong." (For example: if you approach your parents with a question about masturbation and they respond with a lecture about its evils, accept this as their point of view without feeling obligated to disprove them or accept their values.)

9. Use all the information you have. Evaluate the information you received from the person you asked, from this book, from your feelings, and from any other sources you might have.

10. Make your own conclusions based on the information you have, and continue to seek new information to inform yourself further.

Effective communication about any topic is difficult, but because of a great deal of discomfort about sexuality in our society, effective sexual communication often seems twice as hard.

2

UNDERSTANDING YOUR BODY AND MIND

The Seasons of Your Life

In a sense, your life is divided into stages, like the year is divided into seasons. Each season and each stage is separate and distinct from the others, yet all are part of a continuous process. You have already gone through the infancy stage and most or all of your childhood. Thus, you are about to enter or have already entered a stage called **puberty**. Like springtime, this is the season of your life when your body and mind go through an explosion of growth. Understanding what to expect during this period of your life can make it a very exciting time. Not understanding the tremendous changes can result in a great deal of fear and confusion.

Puberty

Since every boy matures at a different rate, puberty will begin for you sometime between the ages of ten

---

and sixteen and continue till as late as age eighteen. There is nothing you can do to bring it about more quickly or to delay it in any way. It happens automatically when your body begins to produce certain chemicals called **hormones**. These hormones, like messengers, alert your body that it is time to change. Hormones are produced in organs of the body called **gland**s. Although there are hormones that are considered male, or **androgen**s, and those that are considered female, or **estrogen**s, every body produces some of each. However, males produce more androgens and females produce more estrogens. The primary androgen is **testosterone**.

You probably have noticed that many of the girls your age have already begun to grow taller and undergo body changes. These changes have been triggered by hormonal changes. Often the first change that boys notice in a girl is the growth of breasts. But as with a boy, a girl's whole body and mind go through radical changes during puberty.

For boys, puberty begins when a thick whitish liquid called **semen** (*see*-men) ("come") spurts from the penis for the first time. However, as much as a year or two before this first ejaculation officially makes you an **adolescent** (this is what you will be called once you enter puberty), your body has already gone through a number of changes that indicate that you are about to enter puberty.

One of the first changes you will notice is a period of extremely rapid growth. During this time, it is not unusual for a boy to grow five inches in a year and to see his body get wider and stronger as his muscles grow at an extraordinarily fast pace. Because of this rapid growth you will probably experience a period in which your arms and legs will seem too large for your body, and every movement you make may feel clumsy.

Dark, coarse **pubic hair** will begin to grow in the area around your penis and possibly on your abdomen and chest. The amount of hair you grow is a trait inherited from your parents, and again you can do nothing to change the growth pattern. This is also the time when your facial hair begins to grow and you will begin to think about shaving.

During this stage of rapid growth, your vocal cords will stretch so much that your voice will begin to change. As it deepens and cracks it will often bring comments and jokes from unsympathetic girls, adults, and even other adolescent boys who are not having as much difficulty as you are. There is not a thing you can do about your voice, or the remarks, except to accept that it does sound funny to others. By late adolescence you will outgrow this change.

Another condition that is sometimes embarrassing to teenage boys is a temporary enlarging of the breasts, called **gynecomastia** (gine-eh-ko-*mass*-tee-a). This occurs in about 80 percent of boys going through puberty and is a result of normal hormonal changes in your body.

Finally, in most adolescents the body begins to produce an increase in skin oils, which clog pores (tiny holes in your skin) and result in a seemingly endless supply of large, deep pimples called **acne** (*ack*-nee). This again is a normal reaction during this period of extreme body changes.

Your Genitals and How They Function

Your body has been going through changes since the day you were born and will continue to do so constantly. Puberty is only one stage of your life, but because the body changes so rapidly during this time it is no doubt the most confusing.

Your Penis and Testicles

Certainly, you are somewhat familiar with your penis and the area surrounding it (the pubic area) because you handle your penis every time you go to the bathroom. Nevertheless, let's take a closer look. First, notice the loose bag hanging down, called the **scrotum**, with two lumps inside called **testes** ("balls"). Actually, each testis is not a solid lump at all, but rather is made up of tiny spaghettilike tubes. If stretched out, these tubes would be longer than a few football fields.

Sometimes the testes and scrotum together are referred to as the **testicles**. One of the things that you may have noticed before is that one side, usually the left testicle, hangs lower than the other. Now feel the area just behind the scrotum. You will notice that your penis actually continues behind your testicles.

Penises come in all shapes and sizes. Like faces, each one looks different from the next. Yours may be wide or narrow, long or short, or even more or less shriveled as compared to a friend's. Even the tip of the penis, the **glans**, may be a different shape.

One large difference in the way penises appear is that some are circumcised (figure 1) and some are uncircumcised (figure 2). **Circumcision** is usually done

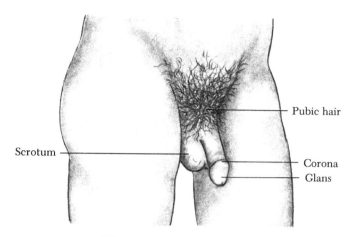

Figure 1 Circumcised penis

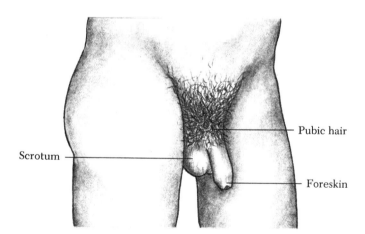

Figure 2 Uncircumcised penis

during the first week after a baby is born, and involves cutting off the **foreskin**, the loose piece of skin that surrounded the glans (the tip) when you were born. This skin is cut off so that it is easier to keep the glans clean and the risk of infection is reduced.

If your penis is not circumcised, you can clean under the foreskin by pulling the skin back and washing the area thoroughly. This is important because a cheese-like substance called **smegma** is produced by small glands near the tip of the penis. If this smegma is not cleaned regularly from under the foreskin, an unpleasant odor or even a painful infection of the penis can result.

Boys and men often seem to use the size of the penis as a yardstick of how mature or masculine they are. In a locker room guys are constantly checking out each other through the corners of their eyes. I could probably tell you a million times that size does not matter, but you will probably check out the other guys anyway. Not only will you compare yourself to your friends, but possibly to a person you've seen in a magazine or film or to your father or to some exaggerated description you've read in a novel. Chances are pretty slim that you would win in such comparisons. It's like standing among a group of professional basketball players: even a person of average height certainly will feel tiny. It is interesting to note that in a sexuality survey conducted for *The Hite Report on Male Sexuality*, over seven thousand American men were asked their feelings about the size of their penises, but "only a few were not concerned with size or felt they were just right."[3] If you insist on making the size of your penis a measure of your maturity and masculinity, you will constantly feel inferior.

Erections

Although your penis has gone through a process of getting longer and more rigid between five and forty times every day since you were born, these **erection**s, as this process is called, often take on added importance during adolescence. Suddenly, it seems that everyone is talking about "**boner**s" and "hard-ons."

Even though it may feel like it, there are no bones in the penis. The inside of the penis is made up of nerve endings and three areas of spongy material. Erections take place when, on signal from the brain and spinal cord, the spongy material fills with blood. Like a long balloon being filled with air, the penis becomes longer, wider, and more rigid, and the skin stretches tight.

Erections do not always mean that you are feeling sexual. Most erections during childhood and even many in adolescence are due to body tensions, motion (such as riding in a car), or changes in temperature (such as when you take a warm bath). As you approach puberty, erections take on more sexual significance.

Erections constantly seem to be popping up at the wrong times, for instance when you are sitting among a bunch of girls and have to get up for a minute, or when you are coming out of a swimming pool with a wet bathing suit on. Julius Lester expressed his feeling about this in an article written for *Ms.* magazine.

No wonder boys talked about nothing but sex. That thing was always there. Every time we went to the john, there it was, twitching around like a fat little worm on a fishing hook. When we took baths it floated in the water like a lazy fish and god forbid we should touch it! It sprang to life like lightning leaping from a cloud. . . . It was there with a life and mind of its own, having no other function but to embarrass me.

Fortunately, the girls I danced with were discreet and pretended that they felt nothing unusual rubbing against them as we danced. But I was always convinced that the next day they were all calling up their friends to exclaim: "Guess what, girl? Julius Lester got one! I ain't lyin'!"[4]

Ejaculation and Orgasm

When your penis finally spurts the semen that announces that you are an adolescent, it will no doubt come as a big surprise to you. This shooting out of the sticky white liquid is called **ejaculation** (ee-jack-you-*la* shun) and is usually the result of a feeling of sexual excitement. Along with this ejaculation usually occurs a feeling of tremendous physical and emotional release called an **orgasm** (*or*-gazz-um) (**climax**). Both orgasm and ejaculation are usually associated with each other, but they are not the same thing. Often the orgasmic feelings are experienced long before a boy's first ejaculation.

It is impossible to describe the tremendous pleasure that accompanies sexual excitement, ejaculation, and orgasm. Like looking at an ice cream sundae, you can only imagine in your mind how good it is until you experience it for yourself. Consequently, all that can really be described in the following paragraph is how your body responds. The understanding of the emotional pleasure will have to wait until you actually experience these sexual events.

As you become sexually excited, you will feel a gradual tension growing throughout your body. Your breathing and heartbeat become more rapid, your blood pressure rises, and your erect penis will seem to get even harder (although not always). Suddenly, from the height of tension, some of the muscles in the area around your penis go into spasms, relaxing and tightening, over and over (these are called contractions), followed by a total relaxation of your entire body. If you are old enough to ejaculate, these contractions force the whitish semen to spurt through the opening in the tip, sometimes with enough force to shoot it a few feet away, or sometimes with hardly any force at all.

After the conclusion of the orgasm and ejaculation, blood begins to drain from the erect penis back into other areas of the body, and the penis often softens. Beginning at this point there is a period of time, called the **refractory period**, during which you will find it impossible to achieve another erection or reach orgasm. In adolescents, this period may only be a matter of minutes, but as you get older the time will gradually lengthen.

This process of excitement, orgasm, and ejaculation can result either from sexual contact with a partner, from rubbing your own penis and body while masturbating (see chapter 3), or during sleep, in what is called a **nocturnal emission** or **wet dream**. Although sometimes nocturnal emissions do accompany sexual dreams, at other times they are simply the body's way of eliminating an excess of semen, which has built up over a period of time. These nighttime ejaculations are usually pleasurable, although for the adolescent who does not understand what has happened to his body, waking in a sticky, wet bed can be very frightening.

Often boys confuse the wetness for urine, but there is no connection between nocturnal emissions and urinating during sleep (bedwetting).

The Sperm Factory

Although some boys refer to the semen as **sperm**, that is not entirely correct. Actually, sperm forms only a small portion (about 1 percent) of this liquid. However, it is the microscopic sperm and their ability to create new life which make this liquid so important.

During sexual intercourse about 400 million sperm are ejaculated into the woman. This may seem like a tremendous amount, but actually the sperm are so tiny that about 120 million of them can fit into one drop of fluid. In fact, it has been estimated that if all of the sperm responsible for the birth of every person who has ever lived were gathered together, they would fit in a thimble.

These sperm look like tiny tadpoles. Like tadpoles, they use their powerful tails to swim inside of the woman's body. If just one of them reaches the egg in the woman's body and joins with it, the woman becomes pregnant. The sperm that do not penetrate an egg eventually die.

The way in which your body produces sperm is both interesting and amazing. To do this the body acts almost like a small factory. The sperm are produced by the testes at the rate of about 50,000 each minute (72 million each day) from puberty until old age. The sperm factory is so complete that it even has a way of regulating its own temperature. You may have noticed that sometimes your testicles seem fairly loose, while at other times they appear to pull close to the body.

One reason for this is because the scrotum acts as a kind of temperature regulator for the testes. In order to protect the sperm inside of the testes, the temperature of this area needs to be a couple of degrees cooler than the normal body temperature of 98.6 degrees Fahrenheit. Consequently, when the weather is warm, the scrotum lets the testes hang loosely to be cooled by the surrounding air, whereas when the weather is cool, the scrotum pulls the testes close, to be warmed by the body.

After being produced, the sperm move to large tubes called the **epididymis** (eh-pee-*dih*-dih-mis), where they grow for up to six weeks. During this time the weaker sperm die and are absorbed into the body. The remaining stronger sperm are then moved by microscopic hairs down the eighteen-inch sperm duct, or **vas deferens**, to the **seminal vesicle**, where the sperm

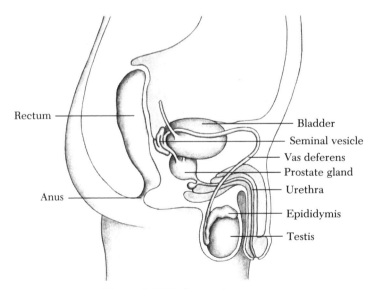

Figure 3 Male internal organs

mixes with the rest of the sticky fluid that makes up the semen. This fluid is produced by both the seminal vesicle and the **prostate gland**. Since the semen is ejaculated through the **urethra**, the same tube you use to urinate, during ejaculation a tiny valve closes the urethra off from the bladder to assure that the semen does not mix with urine.

Feelings and Fantasies

During adolescence your erect penis may often seem like a flagpole, constantly signaling that your body is again feeling sexual stimulation. Your penis and body respond to thoughts, pictures, touch, and daydreams with equal ease, and sometimes you may find your penis hard for seemingly no reason at all.

One of the most enjoyable parts of adolescence, yet often one of the most threatening, is having sexual fantasies (daydreams). You can enjoy the satisfaction of gazing at a girl from across the classroom and experience a sexual encounter without the fear of being rejected. Like a magical adventure, you can have all of the enjoyment without any of the risks.

On the other hand, these imagined adventures can seem very threatening. For instance, it is very common for teenage boys to have sexual fantasies about their mothers, sisters, close relatives, or about other boys. You might see your half-naked mother and feel a tingle of sexual excitement race through your body. Or you might wrestle with your sister and "accidentally on purpose," brush your hand across her breast and find yourself with a firm erection. These can be exciting adventures. Yet, because our society frowns upon sexual feelings toward close relatives, these actions, common to many teenage boys, tend to lead to unnecessary guilt and self-doubt.

Also, because of the taboo associated with such feelings, it is not likely that your friends will talk of similar thoughts or encounters. Each of you will be left alone with these secret fantasies, feeling uncomfortable and strange, only to find out much later in your life that these had been normal thoughts for your age.

As your adolescence continues, your feelings will intensify until, at some point, they may seem overwhelming. It is important at this point that the fantasies and the sport involved in imagining sexual encounters with others remain playful or, if they become real, that they are done with the person's consent. Often, overenthusiastic teenage boys can force girls into situations against their will by getting carried away in a flood of sexual feelings. Even though no harm may be intended, forcing your intentions may be frightening or even traumatic for the other person and could lead to serious legal difficulties for you.

Although adolescence will no doubt be the most intense period of your life as far as sexual feelings, it may or may not be the most pleasurable. If you can separate the guilt and the fears from the excitement and arousal, your years of teenage sexuality can be incredible fun. However, if your teenage years are ruled by sexual guilt and fears, you will have to wait until later in your life to enjoy your exciting sexuality.

3

TOUCHING YOURSELF

When most people see the title "Touching Yourself," especially in a book about sex, there is probably an immediate tendency to think of **masturbation**, which is the act of touching your penis and other parts of your body with the goal of causing sexual excitement or of reaching orgasm. However, masturbation is only one type of self-touching. This chapter is written to help you understand that touching yourself is a normal and natural thing to do and, in fact, may be essential for taking full advantage of your sexuality, both as a teenager and an adult.

I am sure that you never thought of yourself as having been sexually aware as an infant, yet that is when you first began to learn about the sensations of your body and its parts. Infants naturally explore everything they can reach, including their own bodies. It is quite normal for a child to touch his fingers, toes, penis, or any other body part that has a great deal of sensation. Of course, when you did this as an infant you did not identify this as sexual or say "Hey, I am feeling turned on," but it no doubt registered in your mind as a pleasurable experience.

Naturally, people tend to repeat experiences that are enjoyable to them and to eliminate behaviors that cause them discomfort. If there is some pleasure and some pain, then the brain seems to weigh these two feelings and decide whether or not the experience is worth repeating.

It is in this way that this period of infant self-discovery formed the basis for many of your present feelings about sex or about touching your own body. If your parents and other adults around you accepted these early explorations with a positive attitude and allowed them to continue through childhood, then chances are that self-touching is still pleasurable to you. If, on the other hand, exploring your body ended with your hand being slapped or some indication from adults that what you were doing was wrong, then the very natural act of touching to give your body pleasure may result in guilt, shame, body tension, or some other form of discomfort.

Becoming Familiar with Your Body

The following exercise may help you understand a bit more clearly how you feel about touching your body.

1. Spend five minutes exploring your body from your waist to your neck. Feel how warm or cool your skin is in different areas and how soft or boney these areas are.

2. Repeat the exercise, except this time do it to the area from your waist to your knees.

3. Fill in the chart below, putting a check mark next to any feelings you experienced when touching the part of your body listed.

	Breasts	Stomach	Legs	Penis
guilt				
pleasure				
discomfort				
neutral				
other				

4. If you have any checks next to guilt or discomfort, or if you experienced any other negative feelings, think about why touching this part of your body produced such feelings. Where is it that you think these feelings started? What can you do to reduce this discomfort?

Masturbation

Although masturbation is an activity engaged in by a majority of people at some time during their lives, it has only been in recent years that many social scientists have agreed that it is a normal and natural form of sexual expression. For centuries man has tried to stop or limit masturbation, using in some cases "remedies" that bordered on physical torture.

Some of the more extreme remedies involved tying boys' hands to their bedposts or chaining them to walls when they slept; putting a wire ring through the foreskin of the penis or wearing a spiked ring on the penis, both procedures making erection and stimulation extremely painful; the wearing of straightjacketlike restraints to keep the hands away from forbidden territory; and in a few cases, even **castration** [cutting off the testicles] and surgical removal of the penis.[5]

I am sure that in some places these remnants of child abuse still exist, but I hope that, as a society, we have progressed beyond this. However, other obstacles to the understanding and enjoyment of masturbation still exist in the form of myths, fallacies, and misinformation.

Myths and Realities

Now that I have a good knowledge about sex, I can look back and laugh about how ridiculous the prevailing myths were, but as a teen going through the strains of adolescence, I had no way of separating the myths from the realities.

The more ridiculous myths I could toss aside fairly easily. I was confident that masturbation did not cause blindness (although I needed glasses by the time I was eighteen), and I was pretty sure that it would not cause me to become insane or to grow hair on my palms. But the list of fallacies was so long and my knowledge of sex so limited that I couldn't be sure about the rest of the misinformation. It was only later, when I was in my twenties, that I found books that reassured me that there were no known harmful effects from masturbation.

The myths about masturbation causing pimples, stomach upsets, impotence, epilepsy, inability to have children, or decreased performance in athletic events are all untrue. Nor is there any set number of times per week or month in which masturbation is normal or beyond which it becomes abnormal and should be cut off. Today research very clearly indicates that there appear to be no harmful side effects caused by masturbation.

In my own practice as a sex therapist I have found what seem to be two exceptions to this. One is that guilt instilled by parents, religious leaders, other adults, or peers often can cause a great deal of tension during masturbation and can inhibit later sexual growth. Rarely does this stop the child from masturbating, because the sexual pleasure seems to outweigh the psychological pain caused by the guilt. But often the guilt is sufficient to cause the child to become secretive in his masturbation. This in turn leads to the second problem, which is "rushing."

To really enjoy the maximum pleasure from most sexual encounters, two elements are important—relaxation and sufficient time. If you feel rushed and tense during a sexual encounter, whether it be by yourself or with a partner, it is difficult to fully enjoy the rich sensations of your body. Reaching orgasm or ejaculation may not be a problem, and in fact the tension may increase the speed with which these occur (see the discussion of premature ejaculation in chapter 12). However, total enjoyment of your body involves more than simply reaching orgasm.

Try the following brief experiment.

1. Find a watch with a second hand.

2. Spend *exactly* ten seconds exploring the sensations of your arm from your wrist to your elbow. Feel the temperature of your skin, the sensation of touching the hairs on your arm lightly, and what rubbing your nails along your arm is like.

3. When you have completed this, find a place where there is a relaxed atmosphere and where you can be undisturbed for a few minutes, and repeat the touching. This time, however, do it for about thirty seconds to a minute and forget about using the watch. Again, concentrate on all of the various sensations. Feel the temperature of your skin, the sensations of your arm hairs, and your nails against your skin.

4. When this has been completed, do it one more time, but this time in front of a television, and try to concentrate on the TV program.

The point of this exercise is to demonstrate that distractions, whether they be time limits, listening for voices, or fearing someone will interrupt your self-touching, make it much more difficult to truly experience the pleasures of your body. This is not to imply that in order to be enjoyable masturbation needs to involve a totally relaxed exploration of your full body every time. Certainly, there will be experiences when a race against time may be fun, or when the thought of a parent walking in on your masturbation may add an element of excitement that you would not get from taking your time. However, always masturbating under an atmosphere that is tense and rushed may lead to sexual problems, such as premature ejaculation, when you become an adult.

Benefits

Masturbation seems to fulfill two needs that are very important in promoting sexual growth. First, it gives you an opportunity to explore not only your penis and genital area, but also the sensations of your entire body. It is a chance for you to find out where and how you like to be touched. In this way you will find that your needs and sensitivities change from day to day and even from second to second. Whereas one moment you may enjoy vigorous rubbing, the next moment your desire may be for gentle stroking. You will become familiar with different ways of touching your body and new areas of incredible sensitivity.

Consequently, masturbation becomes a rehearsal, in a sense, for later sexual encounters with a partner, a rehearsal during which you can feel safe in the knowledge that you can experiment as you wish without feeling pressured by another person's presence. Later, it will be considerably easier to share with a sex partner your needs and wants, thus removing from them the burden of trying to guess how you enjoy being touched. In my role as a sex therapist I see a large number of men who find it impossible to describe how they like to have their bodies touched, simply because they really do not know.

The second reason why masturbation can be important is because it is a safe and enjoyable way of releasing sexual tensions. Either when you do not have a partner or when you simply want to enjoy your own body without the complications of being involved in a sexual encounter with another person, masturbation can be a satisfactory release.

Finally, when combined with fantasy, masturbation seems to be a way in which boys prepare for their future role as a lover, in this way allowing them to feel more secure in their masculine role. The additional familiarity with their penis and the rest of their body, as well as the knowledge that they can now reach orgasm and ejaculation, makes them more confident that they are one step closer to manhood.

Sometimes men use masturbation as a substitute for intercourse, while at other times it is used as something that is enjoyable for its own sake. A recent survey by Shere Hite found that "almost all men, whether married or single, with or without an active sex life,

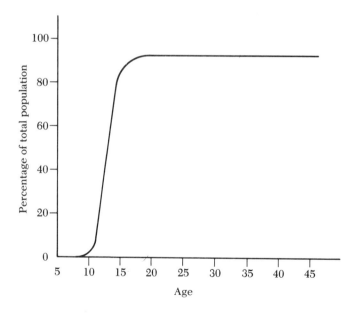

Percentage of men who have masturbated by a certain age
Data from Kinsey, *Sexual Behavior of the Human Male* (1948), page 502.

said they made masturbation a regular part of their lives."[6] This also was borne out by the research of Alfred Kinsey in the 1940s. The preceding chart illustrates clearly, according to Kinsey's figures, the large percentage of men who have masturbated by various ages during their lives.[7]

On the other hand, Ms. Hite reports:

Most men felt guilty and inadequate about masturbating, at the very same time that they enjoyed it tremendously (many had their strongest orgasms, physically, during masturbation), and seemed to have a great sense of freedom and fun while doing it. Most men seemed to feel freer to stimulate themselves in ways they liked, and to experiment, than at other times—to simply play around and have a good time with their bodies. Almost no men told anyone else that they did this.[8]

It seems unfortunate that so many men feel it necessary to maintain masturbation as their personal secret. Certainly the desire for privacy during sex play is understandable, but privacy and secrecy are not the same thing. The need for secrecy stems from a desire to hide what you are doing, often from a sense that what you are doing is evil or shameful. Privacy is simply the need to experience the event without the pressure of others to clutter the experience. It is sad, however, that even though masturbation is a normal and natural event enjoyed by a large majority of boys and men, it often still remains as a personal secret and is frequently accompanied by needless feelings of guilt and shame.

Masturbation Is Not for Everyone

Masturbation is not for everyone! Because of certain religious prohibitions, parental restrictions, or other personal pressures, the guilt associated with touching your penis for the purpose of pleasuring yourself may bring more conflict than enjoyment. Consequently, masturbation may cause more of a problem for you than a pleasure. If this is the case, now may not be a comfortable time to experiment. Rather it might be wise to postpone this part of the sexual process until a time when it feels right for you. You don't need to make up a reason to yourself for not masturbating. When and if you are ready, you can begin. It may be that you will never reach a point of feeling comfortable with masturbation as a form of sexual satisfaction for yourself. This too is all right. Becoming familiar with your body's sensations can also be accomplished by a patient trial-and-error learning process in your relationships with others. Also, the sexual tensions your body might ordinarily release through masturbation can be relieved either in these relationships or automatically through nocturnal emissions (wet dreams).

Whether or not to masturbate, or where and when to masturbate, are two important considerations you will have to face as you mature physically and emotionally. These are not decisions you must make now, nor are these decisions unchangeable. They are decisions that you will be evaluating continually through your entire life.

If you decide that masturbation is something you wish to explore, it can be an enjoyable and rewarding process for you. If it becomes work or a constant struggle, however, then the circumstances of your self-touching need to be evaluated.

A Guide to Self-Touching and Masturbation

No one can instruct you on the best way to masturbate or on the best way to touch yourself. You are an individual, different from all others. Not everyone likes to be touched in the same ways or the same places. You are the expert on your body. This book can only advise you on how other people stimulate (this means to arouse a feeling) themselves or help you find out more about your own particular likes and needs.

Boys and men have many ways of masturbating, but most use some variation of stimulating the shaft and head of the penis. Often it involves a stroking of the shaft, increasing in speed and vigor as sexual tension increases throughout the body. This may be where the slang term "**jerking off**" originated. For others, masturbation may involve a gentle touching of the sensitive glans with the hands or fingers. Or, in the case of uncircumcised men, the glans may be stimulated by sliding the foreskin back and forth. Still others stimulate the penis without ever using the hand, choosing instead to rub the penis against a bed, pillow, or floor.

In addition to stimulation of the penis, other areas of the body are sometimes also stimulated. Among these areas are the testicles, the area between the testicles and the **anus**, the anus itself, and the nipples. Sometimes, the entire body is caressed, as is done in foreplay (see chapter 6).

It should be noted that variations of masturbation that in any way involve the breaking of the skin or the insertion of anything into the tip of the penis are extremely unsafe and may result in serious bodily injury.

If you choose to masturbate, the following is a guide to help you explore the sensations of your body and to maximize the experience for yourself.

1. Choose a time and place in which you know you will be undisturbed for at least forty-five minutes.

2. Remove your clothes.

3. If you feel tense, what can you do to eliminate the tension? Lock the door? Change positions? Put on music to drown out noises?

4. Begin to slowly explore your body, starting with the top of your head and gradually working toward the toes. *Do not touch the penis* at this time. Feel the temperature of the skin in the different areas of the body. Feel the hardness around the bony areas and the softness of the fleshy parts. Pay attention to what feels good to you and which areas, if any, bring about sexual sensations. Also note any areas that feel unpleasant.

5. Touch the area *around* the penis, paying attention to the sensations when touching your thighs, and when touching the front and back of your testicles.

6. Begin to touch your penis, feeling the sensation of stroking the glans and of running your hand slowly up and down the shaft.

7. Vary the way you touch your penis. Try different types of stroking, increasing and decreasing the vigor. Pay attention to what areas and types of touching feel best.

8. Begin to move your hand from the penis to other areas of the body and back again.

If at any time during the exercise the touching ceases to be enjoyable, discontinue it. Do not attempt to rush yourself to orgasm. If you do reach orgasm, enjoy it. Feel the sensations throughout your body. *Do not* try to push yourself to orgasm if the touching is no longer pleasurable to you. If you do *not* reach orgasm, just enjoy the pleasant feelings you have experienced.

Additional Variations

Two additional variations that are often used to enhance or vary the experiences of masturbation are different forms of lubrication and fantasies.

Oils, creams, and lotions are often used to make the penis more slippery, thus changing the type of sensation and also reducing irritation of the skin. Almost any body lubricant will do, but to be on the safe side and to minimize the risk of any allergic reactions, **hypoallergenic** lotions or oils, or lubricants like KY jelly are often best. These can be purchased at any local pharmacy. Each lotion is different in the way it feels and smells, and the speed with which it is absorbed into the skin will vary significantly with each.

Fantasizing is also a way to intensify the masturbatory experience. Imagining a stimulating experience or using pictures to stir the imagination can be exciting additions to masturbation. Usually these fantasies are based upon an exaggeration of some prior sexual events the person has experienced, upon **erotic** (sexually stimulating) literature or films the person has seen, or upon a combination of the two. It is this blend of reality and fantasy that seems to make sexual fantasies so enjoyable.

However, as the following actual case history indicates, when the lines between reality and fantasy become blurred, there is some danger.

Ron's first two sexual experiences were at about age eleven and involved him and another boy touching each other's penises, an activity not unusual for boys that age. He found the touching enjoyable and reached orgasm, but did not ejaculate. After the second time, Ron and the other boy discontinued their touching. However, since the sensation of his penis being touched was so pleasurable to him, Ron continued to masturbate by himself. Since the only sexual activity he had ever known occurred with the other boy, he used his memories of that experience as the basis for his fantasies.

As Ron got older he dated girls but maintained his fantasies of boys as a way of turning himself on sexually. By age sixteen he began to become confused. He was attracted to girls and was completely turned off at the thought of actually engaging in sexual activities with boys. Yet the only fantasies that turned him on involved images of sexual activities with other males.

At age twenty-two, after six years of fears and concerns that at times left him feeling suicidal, Ron finally entered sexual therapy. During the six months that Ron was in therapy, he was encouraged to gradually change parts of his fantasies to include more thoughts and pictures of women. As his sexual fantasies about men changed, so did his homosexual fears and his suicidal thoughts.

It should be noted that homosexual fantasies are not, in themselves, dangerous. Many boys enjoy such fantasies. In fact, the most exciting fantasies you have might be those that involve some sort of unusual or forbidden activity, such as homosexuality, rape, violence, et cetera. However, problems may arise if one of these fantasies is repeated so continuously that you become concerned that it might become real. If you keep in mind the boundaries between reality and imagination, fantasy can sometimes offer additional stimulation and interesting variations to the masturbatory process.

Finally, as preparation for intercourse in your future relationships, masturbation can be varied to help you delay the speed of your ejaculations. This may allow your future sexual relations to last longer and perhaps to be more enjoyable for both you and your partner. To accomplish this, rather than continually raising the level of stimulation to the point of orgasm, stop touching your penis a few seconds prior to orgasm and begin instead to touch a different part of your body. When the urge to ejaculate is gone, return to the penis. Repeat this a number of times before enjoying the orgasm. If you miss in your timing and happen to ejaculate before you planned to, enjoy the orgasm and try again next time.

4

TOUCHING OTHERS: SEX AND RELATIONSHIPS

After years of working to become more comfortable with touching other people, it still is not something that comes very naturally to me. I don't feel odd, because the men I see around me do not seem any more comfortable with touching than I am. Still, I feel envy when I watch my son touch others with the ease of an eleven-year-old, and I hope that he maintains that comfort as he grows to be an adult.

It seems almost as if somewhere there must be a set of written regulations for the American male, including such rules as "Hugging other males is permitted only if they score the winning touchdown in a football game," or "Kissing a girl is worthwhile only if it leads to further sexual activity." Apparently the only touching that many men in our society are comfortable with is shaking hands, rough horseplay with other men, or sex play with women.

At the other extreme, I love to watch the excitement of an Italian family hugging and kissing each other. Father and son, brother and brother, males and males, females and females—they do not appear to be bound by those same rules that seem to cripple so seriously many American males. For the Italian male, affectionate touching does not necessarily carry sexual intentions. Whether with males or females, touching for him can be a sign of caring or sharing or simply a communication of wanting to be with someone.

Coming from a family that encouraged only a limited amount of touching, I remember a situation that occurred when I was about twenty years old.

I was close with a friend who had come from a family where touching was natural and encouraged. When we first became friendly he would naturally touch me as part of his normal way of conversing, or, occasionally, he even put his arm around me to emphasize his friendship.

It scared me to death. I was confused because I did not understand that his touching could be just a sign of affection and not of sexual origin. What was even more confusing was that I knew I liked it when he touched me. I considered the situation, trying to figure out if there were some homosexual feelings involved, but that didn't seem to fit.

It was not until years later that I figured it out. I had not learned that touching was a natural and normal way of expressing affection, nor that my enjoyment of his affection was equally natural. Most of the touching I had known was connected with sex.

Learning to Touch Others

As it is with touching yourself, ease or discomfort in touching others appears to be rooted in early childhood. Physical contact between you and your parents during infancy and childhood form the earliest notions of what it is like to touch and be touched by others. Also, the example your parents set by their physical contact with each other influences your later comfort in touching.

As childhood continues, children touching each other becomes a natural part of playing and fighting and often may reach the point where they explore each other's bodies. Because boys tend to play with boys, and girls stick with girls through most of childhood, it is not unusual for a boy's earliest bodily explorations to be with other boys. Although as they mature many boys become concerned with the homosexual implications of such touching, the motivation behind "playing doctor," as it is sometimes called, is often simply comparing body parts. Rarely is the driving force sexual in nature. At some point, boys may even experience some sexual contact with other boys. This too is not unusual and often continues into the early teens. Gradually, due to social pressures and unwarranted fears that the closeness may be homosexually motivated, physical contact between boys becomes more and more limited.

As the boy becomes increasingly sexually aware, playing with girls seems to become more unacceptable, and touching them—usually a way of gaining attention—takes the form of taunting, pushing, or other types of mischievous behavior. Gradually, as the girls enter puberty and begin to develop breasts, the boy's interest seems to become more sexualized, and wrestling with girls or other forms of making contact with the breasts seems to become more common.

As maturation continues, so does the importance of touching. Playfulness gives way to increasing sexual awareness and to a drive that can become incredibly intense. It is during this period of time that some of the most important lessons that will later shape your adult sexuality are learned.

Becoming Sexual with Girls

As you approach adolescence, sex and interest in girls seem to become more confusing. Sexual thoughts and intense feelings seem to be present almost all the time, and the games become more serious. Touching becomes a need to fulfill some mysterious inner drive, and fantasies about kissing and touching girls become important in making you feel one step closer to manhood. The playfulness that was once there between you and the girls becomes mixed with a sense of challenge and adventure.

It's hard to say when sex with girls begins for most boys, because sex really doesn't start at a certain age. Wouldn't it be great if on a certain birthday you got to have sexual contact with a girl? Unfortunately, birthday presents like that are hard to find. Nor does sex with girls begin with a certain act, like your first kiss. Not all kisses are sexual. There is a difference between kissing your grandmother good-bye, affectionately kissing a girl good-night, and kissing a girl with sexual passion. Sex is really a feeling that lives inside of you. When you are ready for it, your body will let you know.

Like most boys, before I ever touched a girl for the first time, one of my greatest concerns was whether or not I would be good at kissing, touching, and whatever else had to be done. For that matter, I worried if I even would know what had to be done! It's not exactly like going out and practicing baseball or football with your friends. Chances are pretty slim that you will find a girl who is willing to just practice with you. So it is a matter of just diving in and learning by trial and error. A nineteen-year-old related the following account of his first sexual encounters.

It seems like every one of my early experiences touching a girl involved weeks and even months of preparation. I remember planning each experience—fantasizing it and running it through my mind a thousand different times, in a thousand different ways. In every fantasy I was cool and I was smooth, and always, I was successful beyond imagination. However, when the dreams faded and the time arrived for me to actually be intimate with a girl, I always felt awkward and clumsy. Somehow, it wasn't at all what I had imagined in my fantasies.

Entering the world of sex must be like taking a spaceship to a strange, distant planet. You fantasize what it will be like when you arrive and try in every way to plan and prepare yourself for the adventure, but when you finally get there you still feel strange and alien in a world where your body and your emotions are unfamiliar.

In a sense, the best you could probably hope for is to make a little bit of sense out of the confusion. There is so much to know and understand about sex, and so many conflicts and decisions you will face, that it is impossible for a teenage boy to feel totally confident sexually.

One thought that may serve to ease these pressures somewhat is that learning about sex is a process that continues throughout your entire life. You will not learn it all from this book or from your first relationship or even from your first ten years of sexual relationships. Every sexual experience, successful or unsuccessful, will be a learning experience.

Making Out and Petting

Usually, the term *making out* describes kissing, touching, and hugging, while **petting** is used to describe the same activities but includes the touching of the penis, vagina, and breasts ("feeling up"). However, often these terms are used interchangeably, so that neither term really has an exact meaning. There are no rules that go with petting or making out, and what you do is limited only by your imagination and the limits that you and your partner set.

When I first became interested in making out, one of my greatest concerns was how to turn a girl on. Every one of my friends had a suggestion: touch breasts, kiss her passionately, nibble at her ear lobes, or a dozen other surefire ways. One of my friends even suggested rubbing her on the side, near her ovaries (I had no idea exactly where they were or why that should make a difference, but I tried my best). I watched movies to get down my technique, and occasionally read *Playboy* magazine, but I never felt like I had the answer.

Only years later, after hundreds of interviews with couples, as a sex therapist, did I finally find the answer I was looking for. However, before I share that answer, it is important that you do one thing. Don't continue to the next paragraph until you have made a list of every technique you have read about, been told about, seen in a film, or have imagined that is a sure turn-on for any girl. When your list is complete, you can continue reading.

There is an answer to this question, but it is one you may not expect: there really is no technique that is guaranteed to turn a girl on. Everything on your list may work with some girls, under certain conditions, but there is no one "trick" that works in every situation. Every girl is different, and what turns on one girl may not turn on the next one. As a matter of fact, even the same girl may react differently to the same type of touching on different days. A girl's responsiveness may change with her mood, the place she is in (the cramped back of a car versus a comfortable couch), her feelings about you, or probably any of one hundred other reasons.

Hass's survey of teenage sexuality provides us with interesting confirmation of this point. In response to the question "If your breasts have ever been touched by a teenage boy, how enjoyable was it?" only 42 percent of the fifteen- and sixteen-year-old girls who responded said that it was very enjoyable. Another 53 percent indicated it was moderately enjoyable, and 5 percent responded that it was not enjoyable.[9] The point is that every girl is different.

As Petting Becomes More Intense

Petting and making out can certainly be terribly exciting. All of the touching, rubbing, and kissing may even result in your experiencing an orgasm—which can lead to all sorts of mixed emotions. Certainly the orgasm feels great, possibly the most exciting and pleasant sensation you have ever felt. It may carry with it a feeling of manhood and maturity and may bring an added sense of intimacy to the relationship.

However, orgasms are also very draining physically and often suddenly reduce or eliminate your interest in any further sex play at that time. Sometimes the wetness and stickiness of the semen that squirts out when you reach orgasm can bring on a sense of embarrassment. In addition, if petting goes on for an extended period of time at a high level of excitement, boys will sometimes experience what is commonly referred to as "blue balls," which is simply an aching feeling in the groin area. Although uncomfortable, it isn't anything dangerous, and generally doesn't last any longer than an hour or two.

The following account is how one adult male remembered his early experiences with petting.

As petting became more intense for me, every experience carried with it a sense of adventure, and most felt like personal triumphs. I wasn't sure what the triumph was all about, but looking back, I think it was a victory of me feeling more like a man. Every kiss and every touch made me feel as if I were one step closer to my goal of feeling sexually adequate. However, I was fighting a losing battle. Always, I compared my performance on a date against my own fantasies of incredible sexual conquests or against the exaggerated stories of my friends. I always felt one step behind.

There is an important lesson here, one that will be repeated a number of times throughout this book (unfortunately, however, it was not until long after my teen years that I understood it): *As long as you compare your actual sexual performance against that of your fantasies, or against what you believe to be the sexual experiences of other boys, you will feel sexually inadequate.*

Making Decisions about Sex

When you do become involved in petting, there will be all sorts of forces pushing you to go further or warning that you have gone too far already. It's like having a dozen tiny voices inside telling you what to do. Your parents may give you one set of guidelines, your friends another. Your church may influence you in one direction, and the books you read or movies you see may push you in another. Often it feels like a war within; your body pushing you one way, your mind another. These pressures are not ones that can be completely eliminated. In fact, they will be the forces that determine how you handle yourself sexually. Whether you choose to accept what these influences say, reject them, or rebel against them, they will in some ways continue to affect your sexual growth.

Making decisions about how far to go in petting becomes particularly difficult as you become more sexually excited. When you are in the middle of a sexual experience you may feel like you are being carried away by a team of thundering horses. Not only is it hard to pull in on the reins and stop the horses, but you are not even sure that you really want to.

This is even further complicated by confusing emotions. Separating sensations of physical attraction from emotions like love is not easy. Just because you like a girl, feel sexually attracted to her, and enjoy being with her, doesn't mean that you are in love with her. Some people feel like they need to be in love to enjoy sex. Some people can enjoy sex if they simply care about the other person. For others, sex can be enjoyed as a physical act, without feeling anything emotional toward the other person. You will have to set up your own guidelines as to what importance love and other emotions will play in your sexual relationships. Be aware also that the guidelines you set will most likely change with age. One thing, however, is clear: love and sexual attraction are not the same thing.

Responsibilities Go with the Fun

The excitement of petting can be so overwhelming that it is easy to overlook some important responsibilities that go with the sexual experience.

One caution during petting is not to push a girl further than she is willing to go, and likewise, not to let yourself be pushed into actions you will later regret. Each person not only has the right to say no and to set limits, but each of you actually has a responsibility to set those boundaries. To force a partner into sexual acts that he or she is not willing to freely participate in will result in both of you being uncomfortable and may very well jeopardize your relationship. Remember, just because one partner is at the height of sexual excitement doesn't mean that the other partner is obligated to go further than he or she is willing. Each partner's first responsibility is to him- or herself.

Another responsibility that may seem trivial, but might very well cost you a relationship if not observed, is that both partners have a responsibility for maintaining their personal cleanliness. Sex involves a great deal of physical closeness, and as such, body odors and mouth odors can be big turn-offs. It probably won't be necessary to be squeaky clean every time you get together, but a sincere effort at good hygiene may save you from chasing girls away.

Even during petting it is possible for a girl to get pregnant or for a disease to be transmitted, without ever having intercourse. Pregnancy can occur if the boy ejaculates and any semen is accidentally carried from his penis to the vaginal opening. Be especially cautious once you "come" to avoid accidentally rubbing your body against her vagina or getting the semen on your finger and carrying it to the vaginal opening. All it takes is one small drop of sperm to get a girl pregnant. Likewise, all it takes is one contact to be exposed to some sexually transmitted disease.

Before you and your partner engage in touching each other's *genitals* (external sex organs), make sure you understand all of the information in the following chapter about how a pregnancy occurs and how to prevent one, and also the information in chapters 8 and 14 about sexually transmitted diseases, AIDS, and "safer" sex.

5

CONCEPTION AND CONTRACEPTION

For most teenage boys, the object of sex is adventure, love, curiosity. The last thing most adolescents want is a child. If you are going to protect against the possibility of a **pregnancy**, it is important for you to understand how a child is conceived. Besides, one of these days you may decide to have some children of your own.

The process of having children usually begins with **sexual intercourse**. The male's erect penis enters the female's vagina and moves in and out until he ejaculates, releasing millions of sperm in a whitish liquid called semen. On rare occasions, women have become pregnant without fully engaging in intercourse, when in some way sperm was accidentally carried to the opening of the vagina. The microscopic sperm propel themselves with their tails, swimming their way up the vagina, through the **cervix** (the opening to the uterus) into the uterus, and finally, all the way into the fallopian tubes. If the woman has recently released an **ovum** (egg), which she does about once every twenty-eight

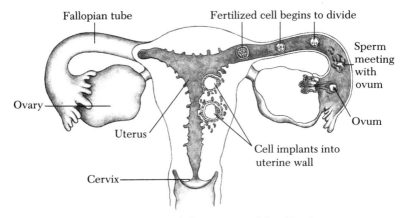

Figure 4 Uterus and the process of fertilization

Ovum released through wall of ovary into fallopian
tube is later penetrated by one sperm cell.

days, and it is still present in the tubes, a sperm may
enter the egg and result in **fertilization** of the egg. This
is **conception** (figure 4). At this point the woman is
pregnant. All it takes is one sperm and one egg. Since
sperm are capable of living in a female's body for up to
seven days, conception can sometimes occur as late as
one week after intercourse.

After pregnancy has occurred, the fertilized egg begins to divide, first into two cells, then four, eight, sixteen, et cetera. At the same time, the egg slowly
moves down the fallopian tubes toward the uterus.
Once at its destination inside the uterus, the mass of
cells first attaches itself and later becomes buried within the uterine wall. Slowly, over a period of nine
months, the mass of cells separates into different layers
and parts of the unborn child's body.

Of Rabbits' Feet and Contraception

Since *con*ception is the process of becoming pregnant, *contra*ception (*contra* meaning "against") is the process of avoiding pregnancy. Whenever you engage in intercourse with a girl, there is a good possibility that she will become pregnant unless some form of birth control is used, and used properly. **Contraceptives** are devices that *reduce* the possibility that a girl will become pregnant; they do not completely eliminate this possibility. Since it takes two people engaging in intercourse to produce a pregnancy, it is important for each to take equal responsibility if they wish to avoid conceiving a child. Even if your partner is the one using some form of contraception, it still is your responsibility to know that she is using it properly.

Hoping, praying, and carrying a lucky rabbit's foot are not adequate forms of contraception. There are plenty of safe means of birth control available today. Even if you cannot afford to pay for them, there are many family planning clinics that will help you determine what method is best for you and then give you what you need without a fee or for a minimum charge. (To locate the family planning clinic nearest you, see the appendix.) Some forms of birth control are available at your local drugstore without any prescription, and others will require that your partner go to a physician. If you really want to prevent your partner from becoming pregnant, it is relatively easy to do. Methods such as washing out the vagina with water, soda, lemon juice, commercial douches (vaginal cleaners), or other household products are *not* adequate to prevent pregnancy and can be dangerous. In fact, under certain circumstances these products can increase the risk of pregnancy or can lead to vaginal infections. The same can be said for plastic bags, plastic wrap, or any other homemade devices. *Home remedies are not safe.*

One method of birth control that is frequently misused by teenagers is called the **rhythm method**. Although with adults this method can be somewhat effective in avoiding pregnancies if used correctly, the rhythm method is not recommended for teenagers. This method is based upon the fact that most women produce only one egg about every twenty-eight days (this time period is called a **menstrual cycle**), and thus, there are only a few days every month when a woman is capable of becoming pregnant.

While this is true, trying to time when a girl is **fertile** (capable of becoming pregnant) is like playing Russian roulette. Most teenage girls vary tremendously in their menstrual cycles, and, consequently, figuring out a time when they are "safe" is pure guesswork. Even those girls who tend to be fairly regular in their periods may experience a change in their cycles due to illness, tension, or other reasons. Secondly, as mentioned previously, sperm have been found to live in a woman's body for up to a week after intercourse. Consequently, even if you engage in intercourse five or six days before a girl ovulates (produces an egg), it is possible for her to become pregnant. Finally, sometimes in the heat of passion, it may become difficult for a couple to keep from having intercourse, even though they have previously decided that it is not a "safe" time of the month. Consequently, even under the best of circumstances, the rhythm method is a very risky form of birth control.

If you and your partner do choose the rhythm method, do so only after the two of you consult with a physician or family planning clinic. The old joke is true: "What do you call a male who uses the rhythm method of birth control?" The answer: A father!

Probably the most misunderstood means of birth control among teenage boys is called **coitus interruptus** (koh-*ih*-tuss in-ter-*rup*-tus). In this method, the boy pulls out his penis just before he ejaculates. This method is based on the *false* notion that sperm only come out of the penis during ejaculation and orgasm. *This is not true.* Some sperm will be released by the penis during the process of intercourse, before ejaculation. For you to pull out at the end does not change the fact that you have already released thousands of tiny sperm, any one of which can cause a pregnancy.

The time to understand the facts about birth control is *before* your first sexual experiences with a partner. Read the following section carefully, so that you understand the benefits and risks of the different means of birth control. Especially important in the next section is the portion about condoms. Because condoms are the only means of birth control that a boy can use by himself, and because they are vital in avoiding sexually transmitted diseases (VD), an understanding of their proper use may make your sexual experiences safer and more fulfilling.

The Condom

I remember carrying a **condom** ("rubber," "prophylactic," "sheath," "bag") in my wallet for years before I ever had a chance to experience intercourse with a girl. I knew that I had no use for it and probably wouldn't for years, but it was like carrying a trophy in my hip pocket. Little did I know that by carrying the condom in my wallet, I was making it practically useless. Condoms react poorly to heat, even body heat, and become "stale." Consequently, the one you carry in your wallet or in the glove compartment of your car may be a good status symbol, but it may not provide you adequate protection during intercourse.

The purpose of the condom is to act like a bag, collecting all of the semen and preventing it from entering the vagina. In addition to being a good contraceptive device, condoms are essential in protecting you against sexually transmitted diseases. For this reason, even if your partner is using another form of birth control, it is essential that you use a condom.

Since the expected failure rate for condoms over a one-year period of time is about 10 percent, it is a good idea to use a contraceptive foam containing at least 5% nonoxynol-9. This should reduce the failure rate by half, and give you added protection against both accidental pregnancy and AIDS. Failures for condoms usually result from them bursting during intercourse or from them slipping off after you ejaculate. If a condom happens to break during intercourse, use contraceptive foam immediately. It is of course much better to put it in before intercourse, but a late application is better than nothing.

Condoms are sold in any drugstore and most supermarkets. No prescription is necessary to purchase condoms. It may feel awkward the first time you pay for them at the cash register, but it's a small price to pay to protect yourself and your partner. Since some condoms are dated, check to make sure that they are not more than one and a half years old.

Condoms come in different colors, textures, and with or without lubrication. The lubricated ones seem to break less often. Sold in packs of three or more, each condom is usually wrapped individually in foil. After unwrapping it, take the rolled-up condom and roll it onto your erect penis. Never put on a condom before a date or put it on a limp penis, and never unroll the condom and try to stretch it over the penis. Some condoms come with special reservoir tips to hold the semen after you come. If yours doesn't have this kind of tip, leave about one-half-inch of room between the tip of the condom and the tip of the penis.

To prevent the condom from slipping after ejaculation, *hold on to the condom as you withdraw the penis from the vagina.* Immediately throw the condom away, but be careful not to place the penis near the vagina. There will still be some sperm on the tip of the penis, and even one drop can cause pregnancy. For this reason, wash and dry your penis before approaching your partner again. If you want to have intercourse another time, use a fresh condom. (See figure 5.)

Condoms are usually made of a thin latex or animal membrane. Since latex condoms are thought to be more effective in preventing AIDS than animal membrane condoms, always use latex condoms if you have the choice. However, never use any lubricant with an oil base, such as petroleum jelly (Vaseline) or baby oil, either on the penis or in the vagina, when using a latex condom. The oil will cause the latex to deteriorate, thus causing the condom to leak.

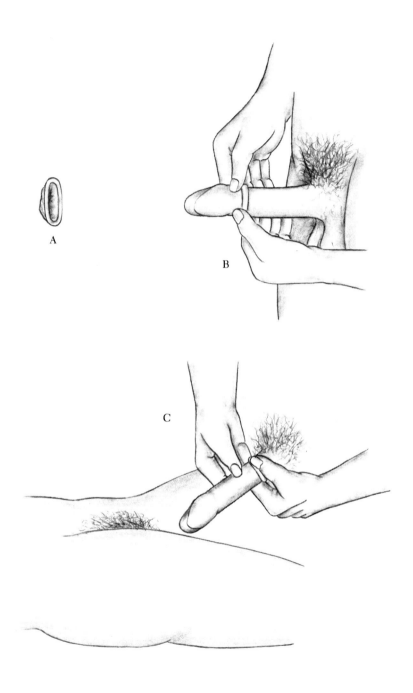

A

B

C

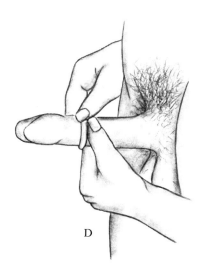

D

Figure 5 How to use a condom

(A) Take the rolled condom. (B) Unroll condom onto erect penis, leaving room at the tip for the semen to accumulate. (C) After intercourse, hold condom while withdrawing penis from the vagina. (D) Remove condom from penis while away from partner's vagina. (E) Dry penis and discard used condom before reapproaching partner.

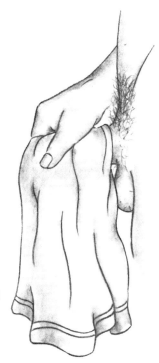

E

Contraceptive Foams, Jellies, and Creams

Contraceptive foams, jellies, and creams are all products that are used by the female partner. Each is inserted into the vagina, where it forms a chemical barrier that kills sperm on contact. Like condoms, each of these products is available in a drugstore or supermarket, and requires no prescription to be purchased.

Foams are generally acknowledged to be a more effective means of birth control than either jellies or creams, but even at that, they still have a failure rate

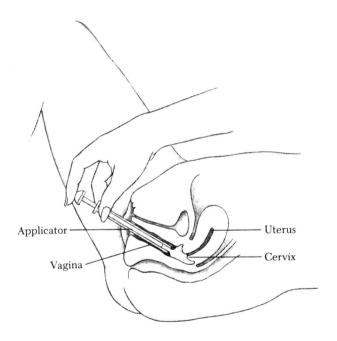

Figure 6 How foam is inserted into the vagina

of about 16 percent over a one-year period. As mentioned previously, when used in conjunction with a condom, the failure rate of the combination is only 5 percent.

Each type of foam comes with its own instructions, which should be followed exactly. Generally, the container is first shaken and then the foam is squirted into a plastic applicator. When the applicator is full it is inserted into the vagina and the foam is released with a plastic plunger (figure 6). Foam should never be inserted more than fifteen minutes before having intercourse.

To reduce the risk of contracting the AIDS virus, always use a foam containing at least 5% nonoxynol-9.

The Diaphragm

The **diaphragm** is a cup made of thin rubber, which is placed over the female's cervix (see figure 7) to prevent the sperm from traveling far enough into the woman's body to cause pregnancy. The diaphragm should be used with a **spermicide**, cream or jelly, which serves to hold it in place and at the same time kills the sperm. The diaphragm must be kept in place for eight or more hours after intercourse so that all the sperm are dead before it is removed. When used consistently over a one-year period of time, diaphragms result in pregnancies about 10 percent of the time. However, to obtain adequate protection the female should have a thorough understanding of how the device is used. She must check the diaphragm carefully for holes before insertion and make sure that it is in place behind the pubic bone and over the cervix after insertion. If a couple decides to have intercourse a sec-

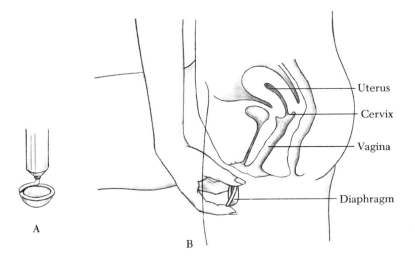

Uterus

Cervix

Vagina

Diaphragm

A

B

(A) Contraceptive jelly is placed inside the cup and on the rim. (B) Diaphragm is squeezed and inserted into the vagina until it covers the cervix. (C) Diaphragm is placed over the cervix and is checked to assure that it is correctly in place.

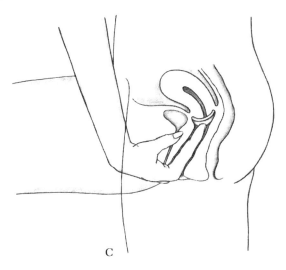

C

Figure 7 How a diaphragm is inserted into the vagina

ond time, it is important that more cream or jelly be added with a special applicator, without removing or displacing the diaphragm.

Diaphragms must be fitted individually for each female, and thus can be obtained only with a doctor's prescription. In girls who are still growing or who change weight rapidly, the fit of the diaphragm should be checked regularly. A girl should never use a diaphragm that belongs to someone else.

The Pill

No doubt the most publicized of all birth control methods is the **birth control pill (oral contraceptive)**. Currently the only oral contraceptives commercially available in the United States are for women, although some day there are likely to be pills available for men to use. Birth control pills are actually a preparation of synthetic female hormones, which prevents the woman from releasing an ovum (egg). The absence of the egg leaves nothing for the sperm to fertilize, and no pregnancy can occur.

Depending upon the brand of birth control pills, a girl must take either one pill every day or, with some types, must alternate twenty-one days of taking the pills with seven days of not taking them. Birth control pills, if taken exactly as directed, have virtually no failures resulting in pregnancies. However, if a girl forgets to take her pill for even one or two days during the month, a backup method of birth control should be used.

Even if your partner is taking birth control pills, before engaging in intercourse it is important that you be responsible enough to ask whether she is taking them when she is supposed to. Taking a few pills during the month does not prevent pregnancy. Nor does taking the pills after having intercourse.

There are numerous side effects, both physical and emotional, that are possible as a result of taking birth control pills. Consequently, a girl can get them only after her physician has examined her thoroughly and taken a complete family medical history to rule out such contraindications as high blood pressure or blood clotting disorders. One other disadvantage to taking birth control pills is that if exposed to gonorrhea (see chapter 8), girls who use oral contraceptives are much more likely to contract the disease than girls who are not taking birth control pills.

Although certainly the easiest method of birth control, with by far the least risk of pregnancy, the decision whether or not to take birth control pills is difficult for most teenage girls.

Intrauterine Devices (IUDs)

The **IUD** (**intrauterine device**) is a small plastic or metal-and-plastic device, which is placed by a physician into the female's uterus and stays there permanently until the woman decides to have it taken out. No one knows exactly how IUDs work, although it is suspected that the device irritates the lining of the uterus, making it impossible for an egg to implant. IUDs are a highly effective means of birth control, with a failure rate of less than 5 percent.

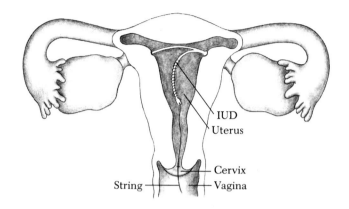

(A) IUD inserted into the uterine cavity

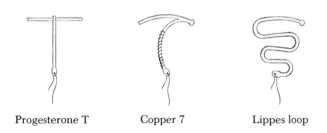

Progesterone T   Copper 7   Lippes loop

(B) Three types of IUDs

Figure 8

Because of medical complications caused by many brands of IUDs, the progestasert is the only brand still marketed in the U.S. Many agencies and clinics, Planned Parenthood included, will no longer insert them into teenage girls.

The Contraceptive Sponge

The newest birth control device available is the contraceptive "sponge." As its name implies, it is a sponge treated with a spermicidal agent, which is placed up against the cervix, in a position similar to that of a diaphragm. Although the failure rate of the sponge is similar to that of the diaphragm, the sponge has two advantages. First, it does not have to be fitted by a physician and can be purchased from a pharmacy without a prescription. Second, it can be left in place and work effectively for up to twenty-four hours. Thus, intercourse can be repeated without having to add more spermicidal agent, as is necessary with the diaphragm. The sponge must be left in place for six to eight hours after intercourse.

There have been some concerns about sponges being related to *toxic shock syndrome,* a dangerous ailment which occurs primarily in young females. Therefore, it is important to follow the instructions for proper use carefully. In particular, the sponge should never be left inserted for more than twenty-four hours and should never be used during menstruation, the first few months after giving birth to a child, or if there is any abnormal discharge from the vagina.

Vaginal Contraceptive Film (VCF)

Vaginal contraceptive film, or **VCF,** is a new contraceptive product that received approval from the Food and Drug Administration in early 1986. The product consists of paper-thin, two-inch-square films that contain a spermicide. A square is inserted into the vagina no less than five minutes and no more than two hours before intercourse. The film dissolves on its own and is washed away with the vagina's natural fluids. A new film needs to be inserted for each act of intercourse. As with other spermicides, some women have experienced minor irritation as a side effect.

Sterilization

Although **sterilization** has become an increasingly popular method of birth control for both men and women, it is not a method recommended for teenagers, except in some medical emergencies. In most cases sterilization completely eliminates the possibility of ever having children. It is included in this book only to familiarize you with the fact that this will be one alternative after you enter adulthood. Sterilization requires surgery, and can be performed on either a male or a female.

Sterilization of a man is called a **vasectomy**, and can be performed in a doctor's office. In this surgical procedure, a small incision is made in the scrotum in order to reach the vas deferens (see chapter 2 for location of these tubes). The vas is then cut and sealed off, preventing sperm from getting through. Consequently, when the man ejaculates he ejects only the semen without any sperm (it looks exactly the same except under a microscope). If the man decides later in life that he wishes to have children, the operation can sometimes be reversed, although this should not be counted on.

In women, sterilization is referred to as a **tubal ligation**. In this procedure, the surgeon makes an incision in the woman's abdomen, then cuts and ties off the fallopian tubes (see chapter 11 for location of these tubes). This prevents the egg from moving from the ovary to the uterus. Since this surgery is somewhat more complicated, a brief stay in the hospital is required.

Preventing pregnancy is not a matter of luck but of planning. There are many extremely safe methods of birth control available for the teenage couple. *Before* engaging in intercourse it is important for you to be familiar with all of these methods, along with their advantages and disadvantages. Sex certainly can be fun, but your responsibility does not end when you withdraw your penis from a girl's vagina. If you have to worry for a month about whether or not your girlfriend is pregnant, or have to make a decision between abortion or fatherhood, the worry can certainly make the overall sexual experience extremely unpleasant. Being responsible about birth control will only help to make your sexual experiences more enjoyable.

6

SEXUAL INTERCOURSE -
THE FIRST FEW TIMES

Your first experience with intercourse will probably excite your imagination months or even years before the actual event physically occurs. You plan it, fantasize it, and run it through your mind a thousand different times in a thousand different ways. Every novel you read and every romantic movie you see seems to bring about an incredibly rich, lifelike fantasy. By the time you reach the middle of your adolescence you probably will have fantasized making love to many movie stars or girls in your school. Each experience feels stimulating and sexually exciting. Every experience goes just as planned, and each partner is everything you dreamed of. Every experience seems so real. For pure excitement and enjoyment, nothing can ever compete with these early sexual fantasies.

In some ways, the experience of intercourse is similar to that of driving a car. You watch your parents and friends drive, and you know you can do it. You understand how to steer the car and how the accelerator and the brakes work. When you finally get behind the wheel for that first time your body feels tense with great excitement and a little fear. Your eyes focus on the road while your mind concentrates on steering, acceleration, and braking. Later, when you become an experienced driver, the mechanics of making the car go where you want it to seem almost automatic. Only then, when your body relaxes, do you begin to notice the scenery outside your vehicle. Your first few experiences driving a car are very different from the ones after you become comfortable behind the wheel.

Similarly, during your first experiences with intercourse, your body will feel overwhelmed by excitement, arousal, and even a little fear. You know that the penis goes into the vagina, but still, your concern will center mostly on the mechanics of what to do. Later, when you become a practiced sexual partner, your mind will no longer be absorbed by the mechanics and you will be free to notice the scenery—a rainbow of new feelings and physical sensations. As with driving, once you become comfortable with sexual intercourse, it becomes an entirely new experience. For this reason, this book contains two chapters pertaining to intercourse: this one, which will take you on a journey through your first few times, and chapter 10, which will help you to maximize the enjoyment once you become comfortable with the basics of sexual intercourse.

Experiencing Intercourse

For most boys, the first experience with intercourse is truly a memorable one. Certainly it can be a time of great physical and emotional pleasure. More than that, for many boys it represents the fulfillment of the ultimate adventure: the one that proves they are a man.

It is doubtful that your initial experience will prove to be anything like your fantasies. Certainly, like any new adventure, the excitement will be overwhelming. You are about to climb Mount Everest or fly your first solo flight in an airplane. Your body is alive with excitement. Along with the emotional "high," your body tingles with sexual arousal brought on both by the thought of having intercourse and by the physical satisfaction of moving your body against a girl's. Your body feels flooded with excitement and nervousness as well as fear and confusion.

Intercourse sounds easy enough: all you have to do is to place the penis inside the vagina. However, did you ever think about how you were going to find the vagina in the dark? It's not a huge cave but rather a small opening covered by a good deal of curly pubic hair. Trying to get the penis in is like trying to feed someone else in the dark. Sometimes it's hard to find where the opening is! Actually, if your date is cooperative, it is much easier for her to insert the penis inside of herself (after all, it's easier for someone to feed herself in the dark).

Once you locate the vagina, entering can be another matter. If the girl is a **virgin** (previously has not had intercourse), then inserting the penis into the vagina may be somewhat difficult. This is because girls are born with a thin membrane covering the entrance to the vagina, called a **hymen** ("**cherry**"). This membrane is sometimes broken well before the girl's first experience with intercourse, but if it isn't, it may take a fair

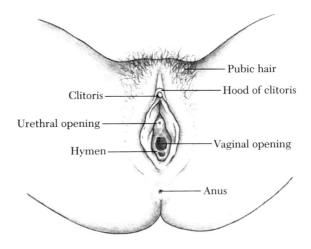

Figure 9 Vaginal area

amount of gentle pressure from the penis to push through it. The breaking of the hymen sometimes results in a small amount of bleeding.

If your partner's hymen has been broken previously, the process may be somewhat easier. If there has been considerable **foreplay** (touching and petting) prior to intercourse, the vagina will generally create its own lubrication, and the penis will usually slide in with relative ease. This foreplay is an important part of the sexual process, not only because it gives the two of you time to unwind, but also because it can lead to increased arousal for you and your partner.

The process of foreplay involves each partner stimulating certain **erogenous** (sexually sensitive) parts of the body, such as the lips, breasts, genitals, and areas surrounding the genitals, as well as various other body parts. There are no rules as to what sequence or with what vigor these sensitive areas should be stimulated. Every partner has different preferences. Being sensitive to your own needs as well as your partner's, and communicating effectively (see chapter 10), will enhance the process of foreplay and the total sexual experience for both of you. Not only does it give the two of you time to unwind and become aroused, but it is also instrumental in bringing about the lubrication necessary for a pleasant sexual experience.

Once inside the vagina, you will find that it surrounds the penis like a warm, moist glove. The vagina accommodates or adjusts itself to the size of the penis or whatever else is inserted. When a baby goes through the vagina during the birth process, it accommodates to the size of the baby. If something narrow like a finger were inserted, it would adjust to surround it.

The two partners usually proceed to move their bodies in a rhythmic manner, with the penis moving in and out of the vagina. The movement may vary from gentle to fairly vigorous, usually until one or both partners reach orgasm. Typically, during these initial experiences at intercourse boys will come fairly quickly, while their female partners rarely experience orgasm. Later, as the partners become more experienced sexually, other types of physical and emotional stimulation usually supplement the sensations of the penis coming into contact with the vagina. When this occurs, orgasm becomes somewhat easier for the female to achieve, although males still are usually more consistent at reaching orgasm.

After ejaculating, you will most likely find that your

erection will diminish and your sexual drive will lessen. This **refractory period**, as it is called, may vary in length from one experience to the next. For teenagers it may often be an hour or less, but as you get older this period may lengthen considerably. However, even with a diminished sexual urge, this time immediately after intercourse can still be a time of great closeness and tenderness for a couple.

Tension and Intercourse

Without a doubt, the greatest source of sexual difficulties boys face during their early experiences with intercourse is tension. With all the excitement, nervousness, arousal, and confusion going on, there is certain to be some anxiety. But much of the tension can be eliminated or reduced simply by dealing with the reasons for it. Below are some of the most common issues that boys mention as a source of tension during intercourse, and some suggestions as to how these might be remedied.

1. *I am afraid that my partner will find out that I don't know what I am doing.* Let your partner know you are inexperienced. If she is too it will allow both of you to talk and joke about your lack of experience and remove a great deal of pressure. If she is experienced, she can lead the way.

2. *I am afraid that someone will catch us.* If possible, choose a time and a place where you and your partner will be relaxed and comfortable. Try to avoid situations where you may be interrupted by

someone (like a parent coming home or a brother knocking on the door) or where you feel that you have to hurry because there is some deadline you have to meet (like being home in ten minutes).

3. *I am afraid she will become pregnant.* Be familiar with all of the birth control alternatives mentioned in chapter 5, and use the one that is safest and most compatible with your particular situation.

4. *I am afraid of AIDS or other venereal diseases.* Use condoms and a contraceptive foam with at least 5% nonoxynol-9, even if your partner uses another form of birth control. This is especially important if you answer "yes" to any of the questions on page 194. This combination will minimize the possibility of your being exposed to any sexually transmitted diseases.

5. *I am afraid I will come quickly.* This is almost standard for first experiences. Don't make any attempt to control your orgasm; just enjoy it when it happens.

6. *I am afraid I won't come at all.* This does happen occasionally, but in some senses it may be a blessing in disguise, in that it allows the sexual experience to continue for a longer period of time. If you do not feel that you are going to reach orgasm, then just enjoy the pleasant sensations as long as they continue. If you start to feel that the experience is no longer enjoyable, then stop. Although orgasm is certainly an extremely pleasant sensation, there are many other enjoyable sensations that will be missed if you concentrate your attention on the orgasm.

7. *I am afraid I won't get an erection.* This too is not uncommon for first experiences. Don't expect

an instant erection; it may take a while for you to relax and get a firm erection. Also, don't be surprised if once you get a firm erection, it occasionally gets softer. Erections do not stay rigid all during lovemaking; they may quite naturally get softer even when you are at the height of excitement.

8. *I am not sure how to satisfy my partner.* In a sense, it is not up to you to satisfy your partner. It is up to her to communicate her needs. Since you are not a mind reader you cannot be expected to know what her needs are. Encourage her to share her wants and needs, and be open to her requests.

9. *I am afraid that something will go wrong.* Don't expect yourself to be perfect. Most likely something *will* go wrong. Many men feel sexually inadequate because they compare themselves against their own sexual fantasies, some exaggerated exploits they have read about in a book or seen in a movie, or against what they *believe* to be the sexual accomplishments of their friends. *As long as you match your actual sexual performance against that of your fantasies, you will feel sexually inadequate.* Allow yourself to be human; we all make mistakes. Use your mistakes as learning experiences.

A Typical Experience

The following paragraphs from Cameron Crowe's book *Fast Times at Ridgemont High* give a realistic account of the experiences of a teenage boy, Mike Damone, as he loses his virginity.

"You're really a good kisser," she said.

"So are you."

"Are you shaking?"

"No," said Damone. "Are you crazy?" But he was. The last time Mr. Attitude had gone this far on the make-out scale with a girl had been with Carol back in Philadelphia. Carol had let him reach into her pants and touch her, but just for a second. That had been enough for back then. That had been enough to make him feel like he and his brother, Art, could really talk about women. But this . . . this was The Big One.

"Why don't you take your clothes off, Mike?"

"You first."

"How about both of us at the same time?"

And as if that made it emotionally even, they both stripped at the same time. Stacy unhooked her top and stepped out of her bikini bottom. She went to sit down on the red couch in the changing room.

She watched Damone hopping on one leg, pulling first out of his pants, then his Jockey underwear. Then he caught the underwear on his erection, and it slapped back into his abdomen. He sat down next to Stacy, expressionless.

"Are you okay?"

"I'm okay," said Damone.

She reached over and grabbed his erection. She began pulling on it. The feeling of a penis was still new to her. She wanted to ask him about it. Why did it hurt if you touched it one place, and not at all at another . . . but later she would ask him that. For now, she just yanked on it. Damone didn't seem to mind.

"I want you to know," said Stacy, "that it's your final decision if we should continue or not."

"Let's continue," said Damone.

As Mike Damone lost his virginity, his first thought was of his brother, Art. Art had said, "You gotta overpower a girl. Make her feel helpless."

Damone began pumping so hard, so fast—his eyes were shut tight—that he didn't notice he was banging the sofa, and Stacy's head, against the wall.

"Hey Mike," she whispered.

"What? Are you all right?"

"I think we're making a lot of noise."

"I'm sorry. I'm really sorry." He continued slower.

What a considerate guy, Stacy thought. He was kind of loud and always joking around other people, but when you got him alone . . . he was so nice.

Then Damone stopped. He had a strange look on his face.

"What's wrong?"

"I think I came," said Damone. "Didn't you feel it?"

He had taken a minute and a half.

They were unusual feelings, these thoughts pooling in Mike Damone's head as he lay on the red couch with Stacy. He was a little embarrassed, a little guilty . . . mostly he just wanted to be alone. He wanted to get the hell out of there.

"I've got to go home," said Damone. "I've really got to go."[10]

There will be no lightning bolts shooting from the sky or stars in your eyes; no ten-inch monster penises as in the sensationalistic novels; no multiple orgasms or moaning and groaning females. Maybe your first experience with intercourse will not be exactly as Cameron Crowe describes in his novel, but neither will it be like your fantasies.

Intercourse and the Law

As crazy as it may sound, there are laws in every state that govern the sexual activities and behavior of their residents. In many states there are laws against having intercourse if you are not married, against oral sex, or even against touching each other's genitals in mutual masturbation. In fact, in some states any person who engages in sexual activities that do not include the potential for a child being conceived is committing a crime against nature.[11] Rarely, if ever, are these laws enforced, but they do exist in the lawbooks.

Probably the one group of laws regarding sexual behavior that is most important to teenagers are those regarding **statutory rape**. As defined by California law (and by most other states as well), statutory rape is having intercourse with any female under the age of eighteen, even if she gives her consent. (In some states a person may be charged with child molestation instead of statutory rape.) Depending upon which state you live in, the age of consent will vary from fourteen to twenty-one, though for most states, it is set at either sixteen or eighteen. Interestingly, statutory rape laws usually apply only to girls under the age of consent. If the boy and girl are both under the age of consent, it is usually only the boy that is prosecuted for a crime.

One additional point of law to consider is that if your

partner has a child as a result of your sexual activity with her, you are legally the father of that child. A court of law can require you to contribute some amount to the support of your child.

Being a Responsible Sexual Partner

Although there is no way to eliminate totally the risks involved in having intercourse, below are some suggestions that, if followed, can make you a more responsible partner and, at the same time, minimize any potential problems for you.

1. Read, understand, and implement all of the items in chapter 14, pages 203 to 205, regarding safer sex procedures. Especially important is the use of a condom and a contraceptive foam with at least 5% nonoxynol-9. Even if your partner uses birth-control pills, or you use some other proper form of birth control, this does not necessarily protect you from AIDS or other sexually transmitted diseases. Do not leave things up to luck. The price may be very high.

There is a myth that a girl cannot become pregnant the first time she has intercourse. *This is absolutely untrue!* If the two of you are not using proper birth control methods, her chances of becoming pregnant are as good the first time as any other time.

2. Know as much about your partner as possible. This again will help you in assessing how risky a partner she is, both in terms of sexually transmitted

diseases and in terms of whether she is underage. Understand that if your partner is under the legal age of consent for your state, some serious risks are involved.

Some Final Notes about Intercourse

One last note that deserves mention is the mistaken notion that a good way for a boy to lose his virginity is to a **prostitute** (a woman who participates in intercourse because she is paid to do so). The belief that somehow a prostitute will be gentle, kind, understanding, and spend time instructing you as to the proper ways of making love is not true. Prostitutes are businesswomen whose business is to sell intercourse. Most of them are not going to be as concerned with teaching you about the finer points of "making love" as much as they are interested in getting you to the point of ejaculation and then saying good-bye. I have talked with a number of men whose first experiences were with prostitutes, and almost all of them reported it to be a negative experience. It is unlikely that engaging in intercourse with a prostitute will teach you the skills that will later help you feel like an adequate lover. In addition, by engaging in intercourse with a prostitute there are serious risks of catching a sexually transmitted disease.

No matter where or when that first experience with intercourse occurs, one thing is certain: it will feel like an awkward experience. You were not born with the knowledge of how to have intercourse any more than you were born with the knowledge of how to eat spaghetti with a fork. You learn by patiently trying, making errors, and then trying again, learning from the mistakes you have made. You will be learning about sex and changing your sexual technique throughout your whole life. Each encounter is a new experience. At the very least, it will probably take you one to two years of fairly regular encounters with sexual intercourse before it feels like a comfortable, natural process, with little or no anxiety. Enjoy these learning experiences without placing unrealistic expectations upon yourself.

7

YOUR PENIS CAN TALK

When was the last time you had a conversation with your penis? If you haven't been conversing with your penis, don't blame it. Penises talk quite well. Don't expect it to stand up and say "Polly wants a cracker," but penises are quite good at communicating. Pretend your penis has a voice. What is it saying to you right now?

Learning to listen to your penis is certainly one of the keys to successful sexual functioning. If you think about this, it's not as crazy as it sounds. After all, you listen to your stomach, don't you? Your stomach tells you when you are feeling full, feeling ill, or when you are tense. I'm sure you have used, or at least heard, expressions like "sick to my stomach," or "my stomach is twisted in a knot." Maybe it's time you gave equal attention to your penis (although saying "my penis is twisted in a knot" sounds very painful).

The point is that your penis is a very sensitive organ and, in fact, may act much more sensitively than your stomach. It doesn't take much to influence the way your penis reacts. If you want to try an experiment to prove this, do something to get an erection (either think of something that turns you on sexually, stimulate your penis, or do something else that you know will bring on an erection). Once you have an erection, think of something that gets you real uptight (a test coming up, something you are afraid of, et cetera). Notice after a minute or two of tension that your erection disappears? That's your penis talking—loud and clear!

Consequently, if your penis doesn't act the way you expect it to, listen to what it is saying to you. If you ignore your penis you could be causing a great deal of needless worry and possibly some serious sexual difficulties.

Both your mind and your body work together as a team, regulating your sexual functioning. If either one runs into a problem, you can bet that your penis will let you know. Because they do work as a team, any problem with your mind will generally affect your body, and any problem with your body will usually affect your mind. For example, an illness or injury (both problems with your body) often will cause you to get somewhat depressed (a problem with your mind), and each of these can affect you sexually.

Physical Conditions Affect Sexual Functioning

Obviously, your body is an important factor in the way you get along sexually. If you didn't have a penis, sex would be quite a different thing. True, this isn't likely to happen, but there are a number of physical conditions that can affect the way you function sexually.

Alcohol, Medications, and Drugs

Just about anything you take into your body has two effects—main effects and side effects.

If you eat hot pizza with garlic and red peppers, the main effects are a satisfied fullness in your stomach and a good taste as you eat it. The side effects may be bad breath, a sweaty brow from the hot peppers, and maybe some gas. You probably know when you order the pizza that these will be the side effects, but who cares. You know it's worth it.

The same applies to alcoholic beverages, medications, and drugs. When you take one of these into your body you do it for one of the main effects (quenching your thirst, getting rid of a headache, getting high, et cetera). But, every one of these chemical agents has side effects. In fact, any chemical that goes into your body has side effects, some of which can seriously affect your sexual functioning.

This may not seem like a big deal, because after you stop taking the drug your body will begin to return to normal. But, in fact, the consequences can be very serious to your adult sexual functioning if you don't understand what is happening to you. Let me use alcohol as an example.

Alcohol is a depressant, and as such it slows your whole body down. Some people report a slight improvement sexually after one or two drinks, because their body feels more relaxed at the slower pace. However, for most people, after each drink the body responds more and more slowly. Included in this is a slowing of sexual responsiveness. For a man who has had a few drinks, it may be more difficult to get or maintain an erection. Or he may find that it takes him longer to ejaculate or possibly that he has little or no desire to have sex. This may not seem like a serious problem, because ordinarily (except in the case of serious alcoholics), his body would be back to normal the next day. However, as the following actual case history demonstrates, when added to other factors, this small problem can change the direction of your life.

Jim was eighteen years old before he had his first opportunity at sexual intercourse. He had masturbated regularly, usually getting a firm erection, but worried about the occasional times when he couldn't get or maintain an erection. He was at a party with a bunch of friends, when one of the girls at the party agreed to have sexual intercourse with him and three other boys, one at a time. What for many teenagers would seem to be a fantasy come true, was about to become a tragedy.

Jim was the first to be invited to enter the room. Not realizing that his being already drunk would make it difficult for him to get an erection, Jim entered the room with one strike against him. In addition, he had a great deal of anxiety stemming from two sources. One, he was worried that his inexperience would show, and, two, he was concerned that the three guys waiting outside might find out if he was not a good lover. With that kind of pressure [see the part of this chapter "Sex and Your Mind"] and his body already slowed by the alcohol, Jim's fate was sealed. There was no way he could get an erection.

The trauma from this single experience was instrumental in directing Jim's adult sex life. In order to calm his anxiety during the next few attempts at

intercourse, Jim drank heavily, again making it difficult to maintain an erection. Embarrassed by these
sexual failures, Jim spent the next fifteen years
avoiding close relationships with women and re-
mained unmarried until the problem was corrected
with brief sexual therapy.

Alcohol is just one example. Serious sexual side effects are just as common with sleeping pills, tranquiliz-
ers, high-blood-pressure medicines, narcotics (such as
heroin or codeine), and with many other drugs and
medications. Everybody reacts somewhat differently
to chemicals. Consequently, listen to your penis. If it
tells you that something is wrong, you might at least
consider the possibility that it is a chemical problem.

Aphrodisiacs

It seems as if man has been looking since the beginning of time for a substance that would arouse or increase sexual desire. In less scientific times, these
supposed **aphrodisiac**s, as such substances are called,
have included concoctions like the blood of bats mixed
with donkey's milk, the powdered horn of a rhinocer-
os, the blood of executed criminals, and ground crick-
ets.

Today, there are some chemicals available, such as
male hormones, that actually can stimulate sexual desire in both men and women. However, the use of
these substances often has serious side effects, and consequently their use is regulated by medical prescription.

There are other supposed aphrodisiacs, such as
"Spanish fly" and similar drugs, that do not actually

stimulate the sexual organs but seem to cause sexual arousal by stimulating other parts of the body, the urinary tract, for one. All of these substances are dangerous to the point of being able to cause serious illness or death. Consequently, in order not to encourage their use, these substances will not be named in this book.

A common misconception is that marijuana is an aphrodisiac. Actually, marijuana tends to enhance the mood of the person using it. Therefore, on a sexual level, its use is unpredictable. For a person originally in a sexual mood, the sexual experience could be enhanced. However, a person in an anxious or fearful mood might feel less sexual after using marijuana. Some early studies indicated that prolonged use of the drug produced a lowering of the male hormone (testosterone) level, thus causing a decreased sexual drive. Later studies have questioned these findings, and the conclusion as to the long-term sexual effects of marijuana is still unclear.

Illness, Disease, and Injury

If you are sick, in most cases you wouldn't expect your stomach to function exactly as it does when you feel healthy. Naturally, your penis deserves the same consideration. Any illness, disease, or injury that seriously disturbs your body is likely to affect you sexually. Having a cold or the flu may make you feel less sexual. Likewise, a back injury or pulled muscle may make sex play uncomfortable and less desirable.

One disease that deserves special mention is diabetes, first, because it is not uncommon in adolescent males, and second because its sexual effects commonly are not known. Some men who are diabetic seem to have considerably more problems getting or maintaining an erection than men without diabetes. This does not happen to all diabetics, and it seems unrelated to whether the case is mild or severe, or whether the diabetes is under control through the use of medications. Rarely is the problem severe enough to totally eliminate the possibility of intercourse. Occasionally, however, if his erect penis becomes slightly softer due to his disease, the diabetic male may panic, causing him to lose the remainder of his erection. Although some diabetic males have more instances of being unable to maintain a full erection, there is no reason why, if they understand their limitations, their sexual experiences would not be extremely satisfying.

Less than 10 percent of sexual problems appear to be caused by illness, disease, or physical injury. However, as with sexual problems resulting from the use of drugs or alcohol, often the panic that results from the lack of a full erection causes more problems than the physical disorder itself. The key to sexual responsiveness is relaxation, and the key to relaxation is listening to your penis.

Sex and Your Mind

As strange as this may seem, one of the books I frequently recommend for men who are having sexual difficulties is one called *The Inner Game of Tennis*.[12] No, playing tennis will not improve your sexual ability, but understanding athletic performance may help in your understanding of sexual performance. In any athletic event, the more pressure you put on yourself, the more difficult it is to perform. It's like trying to aim a baseball at a spot and hit it accurately. The harder you try to aim the ball, the more difficult the spot is to hit. However, if you just relax, look at the spot, and throw, you're likely to come a lot closer. As Gallwey says in *The Inner Game of Tennis,* "*Letting* it happen is not the same as *making* it happen."

Sex is exactly the same way. You can't make your body feel turned on, and you can't make your penis stand up straight. If you're worried about what isn't happening, it is impossible for you to enjoy what is happening. As long as you are worrying about what isn't happening, your body is tense. The more tense you become, the less chance your body has of respond-ing the way you would like it to. It's like going around in a circle. Lack of a sexual response causes tension, which causes even less of a sexual response, which causes more tension, and so on and so on. If your body isn't responding, just ask your penis what the problem is. It won't lie to you.

Of course, my telling you to relax during sex play is like telling you to relax when you have to recite some-thing in front of your whole school. It's impossible to relax just because someone tells you to. However, here are a couple of suggestions that may help if you feel tense during a sexual encounter. One is to tell your partner that you are feeling tense and to talk about it with her. You will be surprised how quickly this can reduce the amount of pressure. Most girls will wel-come the chance to talk about the tension as much as you will. Two, just concentrate on what is happening at that very second. If you are holding a girl's hand and looking at her face, feel the warmth and texture of her skin. Perhaps touch her face and compare the touch of her face to that of her hand. By concentrating on what is happening right then it is impossible to worry about the past or the future.

In a sense, this is the same principle that you use when you escape your tensions while watching a TV program. No matter how tense you feel, as long as you stay absorbed in the program, your body tends to relax. Your mind no longer is thinking about the tension, but becomes lost in the TV show.

One thing that you might keep in mind, especially as you grow older, is that any type of pressure can have a bearing on you sexually. Adult men are often affected by business problems, financial worries, and marital conflicts, which can often decrease their sexual drive or performance. Teenagers also experience lots of pressures. There is no clear research to show whether they are affected the same as adult males, but there is no reason to believe that they are not. If your mind is clogged with all sorts of pressures, anxieties, or bad feelings, you probably will not function as well in anything, whether it be school, personal relationships, or sex.

Another way that your mind affects your sexuality is through moods. One of the things you may have already noticed about yourself is that once you enter adolescence you tend to be much moodier than you were before. Some of this is no doubt due to the tremendous upheavals and anxieties that adolescents experience on their journey from being a child to becoming an adult. In addition, hormonal changes that occur during this period will greatly affect your moods. Occasionally, the intensity of these moods can become so powerful that your reactions may surprise even you.

Sometimes you will feel angry, sometimes sad. Other times you may feel depressed, and still other times you might feel happy and energetic. Your moods may change so rapidly that in a matter of minutes you may go through all sorts of different feelings.

And, with each mood, your needs will change. In certain moods you may need to be alone, while at other times you might wish you were in a crowd of friends. Sexual needs will also change with your moods. I can't say for sure how a change in moods might affect you sexually, because everyone reacts differently. However, as a general rule, people become less sexual as they become more depressed. Next time you go through a shift in moods, think about how sexual you feel.

Although at times it must seem that your penis has a mind of its own, it is *your* mind and *your* body that hold the keys to your sexual functioning. Just as your mind and body have their ups and downs, so will your sexuality.

Your sexual drive and sexual response will not be the same at all times and under all conditions. If you are able to separate out those factors that negatively influence your sexuality from those that turn you on, you are less likely to have unreasonable expectations from your penis. It will let you know how much it appreciates that.

8

SEXUALLY TRANSMITTED DISEASES

From reading the headlines you would think that the primary sexually transmitted disease (STD) is AIDS. Yet, if we listed the sexually transmitted diseases according to how often they occur in teenagers, AIDS would be far down the list. That is not to play down the risk of AIDS. AIDS is by far the most deadly of all the sexually transmitted diseases, and certainly the most feared among both teenagers and adults. However, just because you and your sexual partner test negative for the AIDS virus does not mean you are without risk. Before engaging in any sexual behavior read this chapter and chapter 14 thoroughly. Your health, and possibly even your life, may rest on understanding these chapters.

I am sure that the last thing you expect when you have close physical contact with a girl is a disease. You probably wouldn't be all that surprised if you caught a cold or the flu, but the thought of catching a sexually transmitted disease is beyond imagination.

Think about that for a minute! If you can catch a

cold or the flu from being close to someone who is ill, why is it strange to think you could catch an STD from pressing your lips against a girl's or placing your penis inside her vagina? The fact is that the closer physical contact you have with people, the easier it is to catch certain diseases.

Even today, many people still think of STDs as being worse than the plague. In fact some people have referred to AIDS as the "new plague." They believe that STDs are caught only by "bad," immoral, or sexually perverted people.

The fact is, STDs are very common in the United States, especially among teenagers and young adults. According to the Center for Disease Control in Atlanta, for every one thousand teenagers in the United States between the ages of fifteen and nineteen, there were reported to be almost twelve cases of gonorrhea or syphilis. This number includes only *reported* cases of gonorrhea and syphilis. Many cases of gonorrhea and syphilis are not diagnosed and are therefore left out of the statistics. In addition, many fairly common STDs are not even included in these statistics (because the CDC doesn't count the number of cases for most other STDs). If all of these were included, the rate would certainly be many times higher. Consequently, if you are a high school student and there are one thousand students who attend your school, on the average you might expect that students at your school would experience between one and two hundred cases of sexually transmitted diseases during the four years you attend. Certainly, the rate at your school may be higher or lower than the national average, but the point is clear: all sexually active teenagers share a significant risk of being exposed to sexually transmitted diseases (see the charts later in this chapter for the rates of gonorrhea and syphilis among various age groups).

Early Symptoms and Treatment

One of the unusual aspects of STDs that makes them so difficult to eliminate in our society is that, in many cases, a person may have one of these diseases and have no symptoms at all. This is especially true for women. Consequently, such a person could infect other partners without ever knowing that he or she was "carrying" the disease.

When symptoms are present they can vary widely. STD is not one disease, but rather is a group of different diseases. You can have two or more STDs at the same time. Below is a list of the most common early symptoms of sexually transmitted diseases in both males and females.

> *Discharge*—a clear, yellowish, or milky discharge from the penis or anus for males, or a white or yellowish discharge from the vagina or anus for females
>
> *Burning urination*—a painful burning sensation when urinating
>
> *Sores*—*any* sores, especially in the genital region, whether painful or painless
>
> *Itching*—itching anywhere in the pubic area, inside the penis or vagina, or in any of the hairy portions of the body

Rashes—rashes in the genital area, on the soles of
   the feet, or on the palms of the hands
Warts—any warts or bumps in the genital area
Pain in the lower abdomen or groin—this can be the
   sign of an STD that is beginning to spread inter-
   nally
Sore throat—a sore throat after engaging in oral sex
Sudden weight loss—especially loss of weight without loss of appetite

If you are aware of having any of the early symptoms of STDs, it is important that you get them
checked right away. (The appendix gives information on
how and where you can get help.) If you plan on waiting to see if the symptom persists, or if you decide to
treat yourself, you may be fooled. Many early symptoms of STDs disappear completely or go "under-
ground" after the first few weeks, while the disease
continues to exist in your body, and in fact may be entering a more destructive phase. Just because the initial symptom has disappeared is no reason to think that
it was a false alarm or that your body has rid itself of
the disease. *At the first sign of any possibility of an
STD, immediately have yourself checked by a physician.* Not being examined can lead to great physical
harm to yourself and others, and in some cases can
cause death.

Even if you do not experience any symptoms, if you
feel that you may have been exposed to any STD, go
to a physician and have yourself tested. Do not wait
for symptoms to occur before going to a physician.
Any delay can result in serious damage to your health.

If a physician prescribes a certain treatment, do not
vary the treatment from his or her suggestions. If you

do not trust your physician or do not agree with the treatment, then seek a second opinion. *Do not act as your own physician.*

If you find you do have a sexually transmitted disease, inform any partners with whom you have had close physical contact. Otherwise, they can become seriously ill, spread the disease to others, or even possibly reinfect you.

Prevention

There is no surefire way to avoid getting a sexually transmitted disease. Some of these diseases can be spread by sexual intercourse, kissing, touching, or even just close contact. Consequently, even avoiding having intercourse does not completely eliminate the possibility of contracting an STD. However, there are some procedures that can help keep the risk relatively low.

The following is a "safer sex" checklist. Many of these items are discussed in more detail on pages 203 to 205 in the chapter about AIDS. Read the items on those pages before making any decisions, but remember that "safer sex" involves protecting yourself not only from AIDS, but from many other more common diseases. And these procedures apply not only to having intercourse, but to heavy petting as well.

Safer Sex Checklist

Before Sex:
Abstaining—Do I want to be sexual with this person even if she passes all the items on this checklist?
Drinking or Drugs—Do not make any decisions if your judgment is at all clouded by alcohol or drugs.

Background—Find out about your partner's sexual background. Try to get as much information as possible to evaluate whether she is in a major risk category for AIDS or whether she has any symptoms of STDs.

Condoms—Absolutely do not have sex unless you use a condom—preferably a latex one.

Foam—Use a contraceptive foam containing at least 5% nonoxynol-9 every time.

After Sex:

Urinate after intercourse. Males are lucky in this regard. Since they urinate through the same passageway they use for sexual intercourse, urination can sometimes flush away bacteria before they travel up the urethra. Gargle with salt water after oral sex. As with urination, this flushes out the mouth and creates an environment in which it is difficult for the bacteria to survive. If you have intercourse with partners who are sexually active with other partners, get tested regularly for the major STDs.

Understanding the Diseases

What follows is a listing of the most prevalent and dangerous sexually transmitted diseases, with a little information to help you recognize each one. Although many symptoms are listed for each disease, any *one* symptom can be a sign that the disease is present.

As mentioned previously, because of the current world crisis surrounding AIDS, this deadly disease is discussed in a separate chapter (chapter 14) near the end of the book. This information was placed at the end, not because it is less important, but because information about AIDS is changing extremely rapidly, and placement near the end makes it somewhat easier to update future editions of this book.

Gonorrhea

Gonorrhea is a bacterial infection caused by the gonococcus bacteria and, in fact, is the most common of all infectious diseases reported in the United States. In 1979, there were more than 2 million cases of gonorrhea reported, more than 60 percent of which occurred among teenagers and young adults.

Nicknames
Clap, strain, gleet, morning drip, morning dew, hot piss, dose, the whites, GC

How Do You Get It or Give It?
Gonorrhea is almost always passed by means of sexual contact. Since the bacteria like warm, moist places, they will usually survive in the vagina, penis, anus, mouth, throat, and occasionally the eyes. Outside the human body, the bacteria can survive for only a few seconds. Consequently, it is virtually impossible to catch this disease from infected toilet seats, door-knobs, or cups, as some people fear.

Women using birth control pills are considerably more likely to contract gonorrhea if exposed to it a single time than women who are not using birth control pills.

Symptoms
Males may notice a drip from the penis before the first urination of the day, or a continuous milky discharge

during the day. In addition, there may be an itchy feeling inside the penis, or a painful burning sensation while urinating. If spread to the mouth and throat by oral sex, it can result in a sore throat or swollen glands. If spread to the anal area, there may be a discharge from the anus.

In women, when there are symptoms, the symptoms are similar: a greenish, whitish, or yellowish vaginal discharge, accompanied by a strong odor; pain when urinating; sore throat; swollen glands; discharge from the anus; and a painful feeling in the lower abdomen.

When Do Symptoms First Appear?
Usually the symptoms appear within one to fourteen days, although it can take as long as thirty days before symptoms occur. In about 80 percent of females and up to 20 percent of males, there are no symptoms.

Tests and Diagnosis
In males, any discharge from the penis is tested. If there is no discharge, then a culture (a small scraping of tissue) is taken from the throat, penis, and/or anus. In females, cultures are likewise used from the throat, vagina, and/or anus.

Since cultures are not 100 percent accurate, a second test one week later is recommended, particularly if you have reason to believe you have gonorrhea.

Treatment
Tetracycline, penicillin, or ampicillin are usually used to cure gonorrhea. Follow the doctor's directions exactly. Do not stop taking the medicine when the symptoms disappear. Do not have sexual contact with anyone until the treatment has been completed as pre-

scribed by the physician, and until you get back *two* negative cultures.

Complications

In its later stages, gonorrhea can lead to serious infections of the reproductive organs, sterility, blindness, crippling gonorrheal arthritis, and even gonorrheal heart disease.

Babies can be infected in their eyes during pregnancy, resulting in blindness if left untreated.

Herpes

Herpes is a highly infectious disease caused by a virus. It is related to the common "cold sore" or "fever blister." There are approximately 400,000 new cases of herpes reported every year. It is estimated that about 20 million Americans now suffer from herpes.

How Do You Get It or Give It?

The virus is passed by direct contact with the sore. Sores become contagious about twenty-four hours before they erupt and remain contagious until they are healed (they can last up to two weeks). You can also infect different parts of your own body by touching infected areas. There is good evidence that the herpes virus can survive in a damp towel for longer than one hour. Consequently, avoid using the towel of anyone affected by the disease.

Symptoms

First symptoms are flulike in nature, including achiness, headache, fever, and swollen glands. In addition, there may be itching and aching in the genital area. Later, there is an eruption of painful sores, which may last up to two weeks. During this time the sores may ooze and bleed. After this initial attack, the sores generally return periodically, particularly at times of physical and emotional stress. Although the attacks often become progressively less severe, there is no way at the present time of completely eliminating them.

When Do Symptoms First Appear?
First symptoms may not show up for years after the initial infection, although they may show up as early as within two days.

Tests and Diagnosis
Diagnosis is generally made from a description of the symptoms and observation of the erupted areas, as well as from a tissue culture. Testing is also done to rule out the existence of other sexually transmitted diseases.

Treatment
The only medication effective in treating the symptoms of herpes is acyclovir. However, this is not a cure. *There is no known cure for herpes.* Acyclovir is effective in reducing the symptoms and speeding up the healing during the first outbreak. However, it is less effective in treating later episodes.

Home treatments, folk remedies, and popularly advertised cures have not proven to be effective. Most of the "miracle" cures are based on the fact that the sores will go into remission all by themselves.

The following are a few recommendations that may help minimize the spread and the duration of the infection.

1. Try to minimize the physical and emotional stress on your body. This includes eating a balanced diet, sleeping regularly, and dealing effectively with emotional stress.

2. Keep the infection from spreading by keeping the sores dry and clean. Blot the sores carefully with a towel after bathing, using a separate area of a clean towel for each area you blot dry.

3. Ice in an ice bag can somewhat numb the pain and may keep the sores from erupting. Do not apply ice directly, as the wetness may spread the infection. Some local anesthetics may also be useful in relieving the pain.

4. If the sores do not disappear within two weeks, have them looked at by a physician. Sometimes they become infected with bacteria.

5. Avoid any sexual activity from the time you feel the attack first coming on until the sores are completely gone. Even masturbation should be avoided, so that the infection is not spread.

Complications

Since herpes is essentially incurable, some of the greatest complications come from the victim's fears of spreading the disease to sexual partners. Many people find themselves avoiding sexual contact because of fear of facing this issue.

On the other hand, some people who are affected by herpes feel that since they already have the disease, they having nothing to lose by having intercourse with other herpes victims. This is not true. There are different strains (types) of herpes. Consequently, a person already suffering from the disease can become reinfected with a different strain or possibly might infect a different part of his or her body.

There is thought to be a link between cervical cancer and herpes in women. Whereas most women should have a Pap smear (a test to detect cancer in women) once each year, women with herpes should have it done twice each year.

Herpes is extremely dangerous in women who are pregnant. It can result in spontaneous abortions, birth defects, or brain damage to the unborn child. To avoid spread of the disease to the child during delivery, a cesarian section (a surgical procedure to remove the child) is employed if the mother has an active case of herpes.

In rare instances herpes can cause serious eye damage, spinal damage, or even lead to death.

Syphilis

Although the number of cases of **syphilis** reported nationally in 1980 nowhere approaches the incidence of gonorrhea or herpes (just over 27,000 cases of syphilis, as compared with over 2 million cases of gonorrhea and an estimated 400,000 cases of herpes), the serious nature of the symptoms of syphilis makes this disease one of the most feared of the STDs. Syphilis is a bacterial infection caused by a spiral-shaped bacteria called *Treponema pallidum.*

Number of reported cases of syphilis, primary and
secondary, per **100,000** population, by age and sex,
in the United States, 1982.

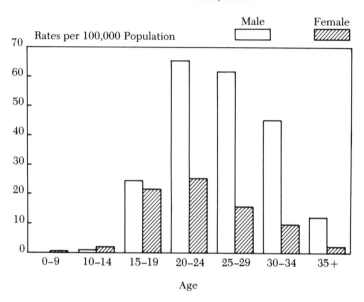

Centers for Disease Control: Division of Venereal Disease Control STD
Statistical Letter, C.Y. 1982

Nicknames
Syph, pox, lues, bad blood, haircut, old joe

How Do You Get It or Give It?
Like gonorrhea, syphilis cannot be spread by such
methods as dirty toilet seats or damp towels. The bacteria live for only a few seconds when away from a
warm, moist environment. It is passed through contact
with the sores or rash—usually through sexual contact.

Symptoms

The symptoms appear in three stages:

Stage I: The first sign of syphilis is usually the appearance of painless, round, hard sores (**chancres**). These sores, which may feel like a button under the skin, usually first appear on the genitals, but can be on the mouth, breasts, or virtually any other part of the body. These chancres disappear in one to six weeks.

Stage II: Months after the chancres disappear, the symptoms of stage II begin. Some people do not show any of these symptoms, while other people show only a few of them, even though the disease is still active within their body.

In this stage, the syphilitic person may develop flu-like symptoms: fever, swollen glands, fatigue, aches in joints and muscles. Other symptoms common to this stage include hair falling out in patches and a rash of brownish-red pimples on the soles of the feet or palms of the hands.

Again, if not treated, these symptoms will disappear within a few months, even though the disease still exists in the body, and will begin to enter stage III.

Stage III: There may be a period of one to twenty years before the disease enters stage III. At this point the disease begins to attack some of the vital organs of the body. The symptoms vary, depending upon which organ is affected. (See "Complications" below for more information about the effects of stage III.)

When Do Symptoms First Appear?

Symptoms may first appear up to three months after exposure to the disease.

Tests and Diagnosis

The VDRL test given for syphilis is extremely effective. However, since it takes six to twelve weeks after contracting syphilis for a blood test to be effective, a test taken too soon may give a false negative and may convince the person he or she has not caught it. Repeat the test after three months.

Treatment

In the earlier stages syphilis can be cured easily within seven to ten days. Penicillin or other antibiotics are completely effective if the doctor's directions are followed exactly. Do not stop taking the medicine when the symptoms disappear. As the disease progresses the treatment becomes more difficult and the cure is more in doubt.

If you have syphilis, do not have sexual contact with anyone until the treatment is completed and the cure is confirmed with another blood test. For safe measure, this blood test should be repeated every three months for one year.

Complications

In stage III, the disease may lead to brain damage, heart disease, kidney damage, deafness, paralysis, insanity, muscle incoordination, blindness, damage to blood vessels, or even death.

For babies who are infected during a pregnancy, syphilis can result in serious physical damage, disfigurement, or death.

Chlamydia and Related Infections

There are a number of infections in men and women that resemble gonorrhea but are not caused by the same bacteria. A large proportion of these infections are linked to a single organism, *Chlamydia trachomatis*. This is a one-celled bacterialike parasite. A group of even lesser understood organisms is thought to account for the remaining proportion. Chlamydia is very similar to gonorrhea in that it commonly causes localized infections in most of the same areas. Chlamydia attacks the mucous membranes such as those in the eye, or the lining of the vagina.

Chlamydial infections are the most common type of sexually transmitted disease in the United States, affecting an estimated 3 million Americans each year, approximately triple the reported incidence of gonorrhea. However, since doctors are not required to report these infections to health authorities, the exact incidence is unknown. They are also a leading cause of blindness in Third World countries.

How Do You Get It?

As with gonorrhea, chlamydia is passed primarily by sexual contact. The chlamydia parasite prefers warm, moist environments like the penis, vagina, anus, mouth, throat, and eyes. Once you know you have chlamydia, be especially careful not to spread the infection to your eyes, particularly when inserting or removing contact lenses.

Symptoms

Very often there are no early symptoms of chlamydia. Individual symptoms vary depending upon the site of the infection, but flu-like symptoms may develop.

When Do Symptoms First Appear

If symptoms occur at all it is usually one to three weeks after exposure, but they can take longer.

Tests and Diagnosis

A definitive diagnosis for chlamydia can be confirmed by laboratory testing. Either a swab is taken from the site of the infection, or other tests can be performed from blood samples.

Treatment

The recommended treatment is with antibiotics. A vaccine to prevent the spread of chlamydia is presently under development.

Complications

Untreated, a chlamydia infection can invade the epididymus in men, resulting in painful swelling of the scrotum, painful ejaculations, and unusual discharge from the penis. In women it may lead to pelvic inflammatory disease (PID). In both cases, it can result in internal scarring and lead to infertility. Chlamydia has also been linked to premature deliveries or spontaneous abortions in pregnant women. Infants born to mothers with chlamydial infections can contract the infection in their eyes or lungs during birth.

Pubic Lice

"Crabs," as it is often referred to, is actually caused by a small insect called a louse, which infests the warm folds of the body, particularly around the pubic hair. These lice can be moved to other sites where there is body hair, by the carrier scratching the affected areas and then touching other parts of the body. When viewed under a microscope, this louse looks very similar to a crab, having three pairs of claws and four pairs of legs. Although the lice are difficult to see, the little white eggs at the base of the pubic hairs are sometimes visible. Pubic lice are highly contagious.

Nicknames
Crabs, cooties

How Do You Get It or Give It?
Although often passed from one person to another during intercourse, it can also be caught from infested bedding, clothing, or furniture.

Symptoms
Usually there is intense itching (although occasionally some people are not even aware of their existence and pass them on to others).

When Do Symptoms First Appear?
It can take up to five weeks for symptoms of pubic lice to first appear.

Tests and Diagnosis
Inspection of the area by a trained health worker is sufficient to spot the lice or their eggs.

Treatment
There is a prescription drug available to treat this disease (in the United States it is sold under the name

Kwell). Also effective are some over-the-counter medications such as Azoo Pyrinate, RID, and Vonce, as well as some others. Besides treating the body, all clothes, bedding, and blankets must be thoroughly washed in hot water or kept from human contact for a week (the lice will die soon after being separated from the human body, but the eggs may survive in bedding or clothing for up to a week).

Complications
The disease may be spread to other portions of the body.

Nongonococcal Urethritis

This refers to any infection of the urethra caused by a germ other than the one that causes gonorrhea. Since doctors are not required to report cases of NGU, there are no statistics as to how common this disease is. However, it is thought to be more widespread than gonorrhea.

Nicknames
NGU; NSU (nonspecific urethritis)

How Do You Get It or Give It?
NGU is passed through sexual contact.

Symptoms
Not everyone with this disease shows symptoms. It is possible to have this disease and to spread it, even if symptoms are not present. When early symptoms do appear, they usually involve a discharge from the penis or vagina, a burning sensation while urinating, itch-

iness around the penis, and a feeling of having to urinate more frequently than usual. Later, as the disease moves into the reproductive organs, there may be pain in the lower abdomen or groin area.

When Do Symptoms First Appear?
The symptoms may appear overnight, or as late as three weeks later.

Tests and Diagnosis
Testing can be done by taking a culture and eliminating the possibility of gonorrhea.

Treatment
This disease is effectively treated with tetracycline, a widely used antibiotic. As with other diseases, the medication must be taken exactly as prescribed by the physician. A second culture should be taken to confirm the disease has been eliminated from the body.

Complications
If left untreated, NGU can move into the internal organs and do damage to the reproductive organs in males and females, possibly leading to sterility (inability to conceive children). For males it can also lead to scarring of the urethra, which may cause problems with urination and ejaculation. In pregnant females this disease can lead to abortions or dangerous deliveries, and possibly result in birth defects or serious disease to the newborn infant.

Venereal Warts

These are small warts occurring in the genital area, caused by a virus.

How Do You Get It or Give It?
They are passed by direct contact between the wart and another person.

Symptoms
The symptoms include small, soft pinkish warts (although sometimes they can be yellow-gray and hard), appearing around the penis, testicles, and anus of males, and the vagina or anus in females. Sometimes they itch.

When Do Symptoms First Appear?
The symptoms appear within three months of the initial contact.

Tests and Diagnosis
This condition is diagnosed by examination of the warts.

Treatment
Treatment of this disease involves removing the warts surgically, by treating them chemically, or by freezing them off. No sexual contact should take place for a week after the warts have been removed and a physician has reexamined the affected area.

Complications
If not removed, the condition can become worse. If passed to a child during pregnancy it sometimes causes growths around the larynx (voice box).

Trichomoniasis *(Trichomonas vaginalis)*

This is an STD caused by a one-celled parasite. Because men often experience no symptoms of this disease, they sometimes carry and pass the disease without knowing it.

Nicknames
Trich (pronounced "trick"), TV

How Do You Get It or Give It?
Since the parasite that causes it can stay alive outside the body for up to seven hours, trichomoniasis is easily passed from one person to another. It can be passed by sexual contact, by using someone else's towel, borrowing infected clothing, or even from infected toilet seats.

Symptoms
Usually males experience no symptoms, although some feel a tickling or itching inside the penis along with a discharge. Females experience intense itching in the vagina and pain during urination. Often the labia become red and tender. In addition, there is a foul-smelling yellowish-green discharge from the vagina.

When Do Symptoms First Appear?
The first symptoms can be expected from one to four weeks after the first exposure.

Tests and Diagnosis
Secretions from the penis or vagina are inspected microscopically. The parasite can be seen in these secretions.

Treatment

Both sexual partners are treated with a controversial drug named Flagyl. The controversy over this drug is because of a number of suspected side effects, including suspicions of it being a carcinogen (cancer-causing agent) and indications of it causing birth defects in newborn babies. For this latter reason, Flagyl should never be taken by pregnant females.

Complications

For males, "trich" may result in infections of the prostate, bladder, and/or testicles. In females it can result in an inflammation of the urethra and cervix.

Scabies

Scabies is an infestation of tiny parasites that leave their eggs under the skin.

How Do You Get It or Give It?

This is a highly contagious disease that can be passed by any type of skin-to-skin contact.

Symptoms

The main symptom is severe itching at the site of the infected area.

When Do Symptoms First Appear?

In someone who has not previously had scabies it may take longer than a month for symptoms to appear. For a person who has previously had scabies, the symptoms of reinfection may occur within a day.

Tests and Diagnosis
Scabies is tested by microscopic examination of particles taken from the infected area.

Treatment
There are prescription drugs available to treat this disease. Besides treating the body, all clothes, bedding, and blankets must be thoroughly washed in hot water or dry-cleaned.

Complications
The disease may be spread to other portions of the body.

Hepatitis

This is a disease of the liver caused by a virus. Actually, there are three separate types of hepatitis, all of which can be transmitted sexually: hepatitis A (infectious hepatitis); hepatitis B (serum hepatitis); and non-A, non-B hepatitis.

How Do You Get It or Give It?
Hepatitis A is often passed by anal intercourse, although it can be passed also by other types of anal contact or contact with feces. It can also be passed by contaminated water or certain types of contaminated foods.

Hepatitis B can be passed by mouth-to-mouth contact, genital-to-mouth contact, or through intercourse. It can also be passed by puncturing the skin with contaminated instruments, such as needles used for piercing ears or for illegal drugs.

Non-A, non-B hepatitis is usually passed by blood transfusions, but can be transmitted sexually.

Symptoms
The symptoms at first are flulike. Included are achiness, headaches, fatigue, fever, loss of appetite, dizziness, and nausea. Other possible symptoms are a yellowing of the skin color and the whites of the eyes, darkening of the urine, lighter-color stools, and tenderness in the abdominal area.

When Do Symptoms First Appear?
Symptoms first appear two weeks to six months after exposure.

Tests and Diagnosis
A blood test can diagnose this disease after two weeks.

Treatment
Treatment for this disease involves waiting it out. Rest and a healthy diet are essential, along with lots of fluids. Alcoholic beverages should be avoided. Physical and emotional stress should be minimized. There should be absolutely no sexual contact until blood tests confirm the disease has passed.

Complications
Hepatitis may result in liver damage, possibly to the point of causing death. Miscarriages during pregnancy are also possible.

9

SEXUAL TRUTH AND SEXUAL FICTION

While learning about sex, one of the most difficult tasks you will face is separating truth from fiction. Learning about sex is different from learning about arithmetic or history. What you learn in each of those subjects is based completely upon facts. In history you learn that George Washington was the first President of the United States. In arithmetic you learn that $1+1=2$. Both of those are facts. When learning about sex it is not quite that easy to distinguish the facts from misinformation or from moral judgments. It might be easier if you learned from one teacher who was an expert in the subject or from one or two books with all the facts. However, that is not the way it works with sex. Your information about sex comes from hundreds of different sources. It comes from your parents, friends, teachers, clergymen, and acquaintances. It comes from books you read, magazines, television, and movies. It comes from serious conversations, jokes, and things you overhear. It comes from gestures, blushes, and from all sorts of signals that are never spoken. As with a complicated puzzle, from all of this, it is your job to separate the facts from the distortions.

Sexual Make-Believe

Without a doubt, some of your ideas about sex are already unrealistic. All of us have some exaggerated expectations about sex and sexuality. You live in a world of exaggerations. On TV or in the movies men are superstrong and women are supersexy. It is impossible to get away from the exaggerations. Almost every woman you see in an advertisement is beautiful, large-breasted, and sexy. Movies make intercourse seem like a natural part of every male-female relationship. Sex sometimes seems almost like a two-person sport, as casual as tennis or bowling. As you watch a movie on the television screen you are no doubt aware that what you are viewing is not real, but only a fictional story. However, sometimes it is difficult to realize that the way sex is portrayed is likewise a world of make-believe.

The reason for these distortions is simple. People pay attention to sex. Sexy girls in advertisements sell products. Sex sells books and magazines. The more exaggerated the sex appears to be, the more people seem to pay attention. Along with capturing your attention, however, these distortions will most likely give you false expectations.

Below are a few questions that may help you evaluate some of your sexual expectations and the sources from which they originate.

1. Do you consider women sexier if they have large breasts rather than small breasts? If so, where did this idea originate?

2. If you are currently dating, do you feel like you failed if you don't "go a little further" sexually on each date?

3. What do you think girls find attractive in a boy? Where did this idea come from?

4. Do you feel you are as masculine as other boys at your school? Where did your definition of masculine come from?

No matter what your answers are to these questions, begin to pay attention to what the sources are for most of your sexual ideas. As mentioned previously in this book, if you compare yourself with the image of male sexuality that is painted by the media or by the stories of other teenage boys, you will certainly feel sexually inadequate. It is difficult enough for you to make sense of the sexual feelings and thoughts that your teenage body is experiencing. Adding to these the pressure of living up to the lies, fabrications, and exaggerations of others can make your teenage years unbearable.

Opinions versus Facts

Even the words people use (or misuse) in describing sex are important in influencing your sexual attitudes and opinions. In talking with others, you will encounter terms used to describe varying aspects of sex: *normal* and *abnormal*, *bad* and *good*, *right* and *wrong*, *healthy* and *unhealthy.* Unfortunately, these terms are overused and abused.

Normal is a statistical term meaning "usual." It is "normal" for most people to put one sock on each of their feet and then to put on both shoes, but occasionally someone likes to put on his left sock and shoe, followed by his right sock and shoe. Even though this person might be considered "abnormal," because he doesn't do what is *usual* for most people, it does not mean he is sick, crazy, or weird. It means he has his own way of doing things. Just because you don't conform to what most people do, doesn't mean there is something wrong with you.

Sometimes words are misused in a different way. When people are uncomfortable about something, they sometimes will refer to it as "abnormal," "wrong," "bad," "unhealthy," or use some similar term. For example, it is not uncommon to hear people talk about masturbation as being "abnormal." Since surveys have shown that over 90 percent of adult men and a large majority of teenage boys do masturbate, that behavior is certainly statistically "normal." What these people mean to say is that they don't approve of masturbation. This certainly is their privilege. However, that has nothing to do with abnormal, normal, right, or wrong. What it has to do with is their personal beliefs.

Many people, while talking about sex, will confuse facts and opinions. If someone says "A girl may become pregnant if she engages in intercourse," that is a fact. If they say that it is "good" or "bad" for her to engage in intercourse, that is their opinion. Opinions and facts are not the same.

Sexual Distortions

In all of the confusion about sexual distortion there is some good news and some bad news. The good news is that your parents, grandparents, clergymen, teachers, and everyone else who is an important influence in helping to mold your sexual ideas, have been through the same confusion you are going through. They have had to sort through all of the facts, beliefs, opinions, and myths in order to form the sexual attitudes and ideas that work for them. Certainly, each of them may have had different pressures than you are facing, but basically the process was the same.

The bad news is that they possibly still hold on to some of the myths and may pass them on to you. It is like the old joke where Johnny, who is eleven years old, is sitting in his room exploring his penis when his mother comes walking unexpectedly through the door. His mother, herself believing an old wives' tale, says, "Johnny, you stop that this instant! Don't you know that touching yourself that way will cause you to go blind?" To which Johnny quickly replies, "Oh mom, it feels so good. Can't I just do it until I need to wear glasses?"

The point is that parents and friends are human also. They too have been taught some distorted information, and they too may sometimes unknowingly communicate this to you.

If a piece of information you receive from one source doesn't match with other information you have learned, often the problem can be solved by going to a third source. Even as you read this book, if some of the information doesn't match with the facts you presently believe, check things out by going to a third source. The Appendix contains a list of books that you might want to read in order to check out any doubts. In addition, there are many agencies listed in the Appendix, many of which could answer any questions you might have.

Self-Distortions

Not all sexual distortions are caused by outside sources. Sometimes boys create their own distortions about sex. The following case history is a good example of how one boy pieced together some facts and some exaggerations and created a fear that caused him some very serious psychological problems.

John was a fifteen-year-old boy who was brought by his mother for counseling because of difficulties he was having with school and with relating to his friends. After the first few counseling sessions, John revealed that one of his fears was that he was a homosexual. Although he in no way felt sexually attracted to other boys, in his own mind John had put together a number of unrealistic fears and a lot of misinformation and reached the conclusion he was "gay." Following is the information that John distorted to reach his erroneous conclusions.

1. Apparently because he was shy and unathletic, boys teased him by calling him "gay," "fag," "homo," or other terms that implied he was a homosexual. Not realizing that many boys do this as

a way of teasing, he assumed that they saw something about him that looked "gay," and began to worry that maybe they were right.

2. John worried that he masturbated "too much." Although John had no idea what a "normal" amount of masturbation might be, he was positive that the amount he was masturbating was "too much."

3. John was shy with girls. Even though he felt sexually attracted to them, his fear of socializing with girls made him doubt his masculinity. He was not aware that neither shyness nor masculinity has anything to do with homosexuality.

4. Although he sometimes had strong sexual feelings toward girls, John was concerned because at other times he had little interest at all [see myth #1 on the next page].

5. John had been molested as a young child by an adult male, who made John play with the man's penis. John decided that this must be the event that caused his homosexuality.

6. Since John's mother was divorced, and since he had no contact with his father, John had no male with whom he could share his fears or after whom he could model himself.

Although John had other problems that required him to remain in counseling almost a year, his sexual fears and problems relating to friends were reversed within three months, after he fully understood how his misconceptions about masculinity, sexuality, and homosexuality combined to cause him unnecessary fears about himself.

Myths

There seem to be an endless number of sexual myths. The following pages are written about some of the most common ones that boys and men use to torture themselves. (Myths dealt with in other parts of this book are not included in this section.)

Myth 1: Guys are always in the mood for sex.

Truth 1: Have you ever just *not* been in the mood for something you usually enjoy—ice cream, your best friend, going to the beach? Sex is the same way. Sometimes you just may not be in a sexual mood. There seems to be a common misbelief that guys always feel sexually turned-on and, unfortunately, that myth seems to get a lot of guys in trouble. If you are really not in a sexual mood, you are better off not even trying. Not only is it possible that your penis won't be up to it (if you try to have intercourse), but, in addition, your partner will be able to read your lack of enthusiasm and may feel like you're not interested in her. You are better off sharing in the first place that you are not in the mood. The urge for sex will come and go. As a teenager, that urge may be present much of the time, but throughout your adulthood, the periods of sexual interest may lessen with age. *Men do not always feel sexual.*

Myth 2: Males are supposed to be in charge sexually.

Truth 2: Along with the myth that guys always feel sexual, there seem to be dozens of similar myths about how guys are supposed to be the first ones to make sexual advances in a relationship with a girl, or just generally, that boys are supposed to always be in charge sexually. The way you handle your relationship with a girl is a decision the two of you will make. However, be aware that if you are expecting yourself always to be in charge, to make all the decisions, and to be the "teacher" in your sexual relationships, then you are taking on an awfully large responsibility. There is no reason to think that boys are more knowledgeable about sex than girls, or that for some reason boys should be in charge.

Myth 3: A good lover is one who knows how to turn on his partner.

Truth 3: This myth is believed not only by many boys, but even many adult men share this misconception. Actually, if you stop and think, it is impossible to know how to turn on your partner. All girls are different, and each has different sexual likes and dislikes. Even if you have a sexual relationship with one girl over a long period of time, her needs will continually change from one day to the next. Certainly, you may learn specific things that she seems to enjoy, and others that she doesn't. However, that will only happen if you are a good listener *and* if she is good at communicating. A good lover is one who listens to the needs and wants of his partner, and shares his own needs. *No matter how much sexual experience and knowledge you have, your partner will always know more about her own likes and dislikes than you do. Listen to her.*

Interestingly, when it comes to sexual therapy,

it is often more difficult to help men who have a great deal of sexual experience than those who have had few sexual encounters. The reason is that the more sexually experienced men often feel that they know so much about sex that they do not have to listen to their partners.

Myth 4: Girls say no even when they mean yes.

Truth 4: This is one myth that seems to get a lot of boys into trouble. At a time when you are feeling really turned on sexually, you may find it easy to kid yourself into the belief that a girl's resistance is not real. However, to push a girl further than she is willing to go sexually will often lead to serious problems in your relationship, and possibly even legal problems if she is pushed too far.

Myth 5: Sex and intercourse are the same thing.

Truth 5: One of the things you have probably noticed about this book is that it does not refer to sex and intercourse as if they were the same thing. Intercourse is only one form of sex. Making out, masturbation, and petting are also forms of sex, not just substitutes for intercourse. Each may be enjoyable in itself, and it is possible that all of these behaviors will continue even after you begin to engage regularly in intercourse. Even fantasies and dreams can be considered forms of sex, and very enjoyable ones at that. To think of intercourse as the only form of sex is like thinking of hamburgers as the only form of food. Fantasies, dreams, kissing, foreplay, petting, and masturbation are all forms of sex that may add interest to your sexual experiences.

Myth 6: Sex will magically cure all of your problems.

Truth 6: Sex is certainly a very special experience, but it is not at all a panacea or cure-all. Enjoying a sexual relationship will not make you more masculine, nor will it cure pimples. As a form of communication, it may be a way of sharing that can bring a relationship closer, but it cannot singlehandedly solve all your problems.

Myth 7: As you get older you will naturally know more about what to do sexually.

Truth 7: Sexual knowledge has little to do with age. Certainly, as your body matures you will experience a wide range of sexual feelings. However, unless you have the facts on what those feelings are about, the feelings will just be confusing to you.

Although understanding these myths is a useful tool in trying to make sense from your own sexual confusion, this is only one step toward understanding sexual distortions. Since sexual myths can only be transmitted from one person to another when there is a lack of understanding of the facts, the only way to fully erase all of them from your mind is by completely understanding the facts.

10

AS SEXUAL RELATIONSHIPS CONTINUE

As you become more sexually experienced, the nature of your sexual relationships is likely to change. The changes are not exactly the same for all boys, but nevertheless you will experience some. When you first learned to ride a bicycle, the awkwardness and the fear you initially experienced eventually gave way to comfort and relaxation. With this relaxation, your mind gradually switched its focus from thoughts of how to control what seemed like a two-wheeled monster, to experimentation—first riding with one hand, then with no hands.

In some ways your experiences with sex will be similar. With each new stage of sexual experimentation, and with each new relationship, your focus at first will be on the fundamentals. After the awkwardness fades, your mind will turn to thoughts of new and different types of experiences. Gradually, your relationships with girls will become increasingly complex and new skills will become more important.

Sexual Communication Between Partners

One skill that too often is ignored as being an important part of sex is communication. If you try to maintain a long-term relationship, clear communication is essential. Communication is the only way for each partner to learn about the other's likes and dislikes. In chapter 1 a few basic principles were discussed in regard to communicating with your parents. As you will see, some of those same principles apply to communicating with your sexual partners.

In any relationship with a girl there is communication, whether it is intended or not. If she pays attention to you, smiles at you, and talks to you, you may understand her message to mean "she likes me." If she does nothing and simply ignores you, you may understand her message to mean "she doesn't think much of me." If you take a girl's hand, one message is communicated; if you don't, you communicate another. In each of these situations, messages are being exchanged between the two of you; the two of you are communicating. *There is no such thing as not communicating.* Every movement of your body and every expression on your face sends a message. Every word from your mouth and every gesture and touch of your hand communicates something.

Nonverbal Communication

Because of the close physical contact involved in a sexual relationship, touch becomes an especially important form of communication. Every touch and every avoidance of a touch sends a message.

As an experiment, examine the following list of actions that might be a part of your relationship with a girl. Read each one and imagine two or three messages the girl might interpret from each action.

1. A gentle hug
2. A lengthy embrace
3. Aggressively taking her hand
4. Not taking her hand
5. Stroking her breast gently
6. Grabbing her breast

As you can conclude from your imagined responses, messages communicated through touch have a lot of room for being misinterpreted.

If each of the messages in the example above could have two or three possible interpretations, then a great deal may depend upon other messages you send or possibly even upon what kind of mood your partner is in. In example 4 above, if the girl is in a good mood, she might interpret your not taking her hand as an indication that you are shy. If she is feeling insecure, she may take it as a rejection. In any sexual relationship, be aware that your touch is an important means of communication. This will allow you to send clearer messages to your sexual partners.

Verbal Communication

Although spoken messages, like nonverbal messages, are sometimes misinterpreted, words are probably the best tool we have for making a clear communication. Yet, because many people are not comfortable talking about sex, or because they feel that sex is a thing that should happen between people without any words being spoken, sexual messages often can be unclear.

It is common, when people think of the organs of the body that are important in sex, that their first thoughts turn to the penis and the vagina. However, as the following section makes clear, in many sexual relationships your ears may play a considerably more important role than either the penis or vagina. Not because your ears feel good during sex, but because of the vital role they play in verbal communication.

In a sense, words and touch are tools that we use to communicate messages. As with any other tool, they are effective when used properly and ineffective when not. If you use a knife to cut meat it works fine. If you use it as a screwdriver, sometimes it works and sometimes it doesn't. Words and touch are likewise effective when they are used properly as tools of sexual communication.

Communicating Effectively

Good sexual communication can be boiled down to one apparently simple rule: *Let your partner know clearly what you want.* What seems like a simple rule, however, can be deceiving. Often couples— even couples who have been together for many years—run into problems because of one of the following reasons.

1. One person follows the rule (lets the partner know what is wanted), while the other partner

doesn't. This tends to make the relationship one-sided, with one partner getting most of what he or she wants, while the other partner ends up unsatisfied. Although it would appear that this would be great for the person who is getting all needs met, eventually the unsatisfied person becomes frustrated, sometimes to the point of breaking off the relationship. *Always state clearly what you are wanting, and encourage your partner to do the same.*

2. One or both partners become comfortable at saying what they *don't* want, but fail to communicate what they *do* want. *Rather than constantly criticizing your partner by telling her what she is doing wrong, give her guidance as to what you would like from her.* If your partner hears only what you *don't* want, she must guess in order to figure out what you *do* want. In addition, after a while it is likely to become frustrating and depressing for her if all she hears is what she is doing wrong.

3. Setting limits is critical. Both of you have limits beyond which you will not go. *Never let yourself get forced into anything beyond your limit, and never force your partner beyond hers.* The following case history indicates what sometimes occurs when one person refuses to set a limit in a sexual relationship.

Joe and Vicki enjoyed their sexual relationship during the first two months of their marriage, engaging in intercourse four or five times each week. Although Joe did not always feel in a sexual mood, he did not want to disappoint his new wife. In addition, he was afraid that she might view his lack of sexual drive as unmasculine. Consequently, he pretended to enjoy these encounters, even though he some-times felt uninvolved. Vicki, sensing a coldness in Joe on these occasions, began to feel rejected.

As their marriage continued, Joe found excuses for not engaging in sex. He sometimes would work late or would pick fights with Vicki as a way of avoiding closeness, but never openly talked about his growing disinterest. Vicki's feelings of rejection began to in-crease.

After a while the couple reached a point of rarely engaging in any sexual activities, and even ceased acting affectionate toward each other. A problem that easily could have been avoided if Joe had been willing to set his limits and say no blew up into a problem that required a great deal of counseling to resolve.

If you are going to have sexual contact, do it at a time you can enjoy it and in a way you can enjoy it. People tend to repeat events that they enjoy and to avoid situations that are unpleasant to them. If you have a favorite subject or favorite teacher at school, most likely you enjoy going to that class. However, in the case of a subject that is boring to you or one in which you don't like the teacher, you can probably think of hundreds of different excuses for not going to class. It is the same with sex. If you participate sexually with your partner when you are not in the mood, you will likely end up not enjoying the contact. Over a pe-riod of time your mind and your body will probably figure out lots of ways to avoid most sexual contact. On the other hand, if you honestly avoid potentially un-pleasant experiences and most of your sexual encounters end up being pleasurable, you will find yourself looking forward to more in the future.

Saying no to your partner is extremely important. However, do it in a way that rejects the sexual opportunity, not your partner. Giving in because you feel obligated to is not a good solution. As mentioned previously, try to let your partner know what you *do* want. Give her an alternative. "I'm not in the mood right now because I feel rushed; tomorrow I think I'll feel more relaxed." Or "Don't hold my hand when my friends are around; I'd rather you only do that in private." Even if it is tentative, give your partner an alternative. Let her know that you're not avoiding the issue.

Sex and Love

For years, various poets, philosophers, and authors have written about the meaning of love. Each in his own way defined love as he or she experienced it. Similarly, you will have to define love as it is to you. Because it is such an individual matter, deciding the importance of love in a sexual relationship similarly must be an individual matter. For some people, love is a necessary ingredient in a sexual relationship; for others sex can be enjoyed without any romantic attachments. However, no matter how you define the relationship between love and sex, it is likely to change as you mature. As with most aspects of sexuality, there is no *right* way and no *wrong* way to view this matter.

Sexual Positions and Variations

There are probably as many different ways to enjoy sex as there are people who enjoy it. Every person has his or her own sexual preferences. Some people find pleasure in a relatively set sexual routine, enjoying sex in a single position with little or no variation. Others enjoy sex in a much more spontaneous way, varying many aspects of their sexual positions.

As a teenager, you will be exposed to many words and expressions that refer to various sexual positions. Some of these will sound rather bizarre and may bring on a sense of curiosity, while others may bring on feelings of excitement, disgust, or various other responses. Whatever your personal reaction, remember that when you are in a sexual relationship you and your partner will be making your own decisions. There is no rule that you must try all of these variations, nor, for that matter, is it necessary that you even try any of them. However, because it is likely that you will hear many of these terms and in some cases may not know exactly what they mean, below are the definitions of various words and common slang expressions you may encounter, which are associated with different sexual positions. These are not the only sexual positions that exist. The number and variety of sexual positions you may someday enjoy is limited only by the creativity of your imagination.

Male-superior position (missionary position): A position of intercourse where the male lies in a face-to-face position on top of the female.

Female-superior position: A position of intercourse where the female lies in a face-to-face position on top of the male.

Oral sex: A general term for any sexual stimulation in which the mouth is used to stimulate either the male genitals or the female genitals.

Cunnilingus: The type of oral sex in which the mouth is used to stimulate the female genitals.

Fellatio: The type of oral sex in which the mouth is used to stimulate the male genitals.

69: A combination of cunnilingus and fellatio at the same time. This position is referred to as 69 because the positions of the body form a figure that looks similar to the number *69*.

Anal sex: A type of sexual contact in which the penis is inserted into the rectum.

Lateral position: A position of intercourse in which the couple lies in a side-by-side position, facing each other.

11

THE FEMALE BODY

To hear many teenage boys talk, you would think that a woman's sexual parts consist of two breasts, a single hole called the **vagina** (sometimes referred to in slang as a "cunt" or a "box") and nothing else. However, in actuality, a woman's body is much more complex than that. To make it easier for you to understand and visualize, this chapter will divide the woman's sexual organs into two parts, those that can be seen outside of her body, and those that are inside of her body. In addition there will be a separate portion of this chapter explaining the breasts, and one that explains a girl's "periods" and what is known as the menstrual cycle.

Outer Genitals

The external sexual organs of a girl's body are referred to as the **vulva.** Figure 10 shows how the vulva looks normally and what it looks like when it is spread apart. Although all girls have the same basic parts to their bodies, no two girls look exactly alike around their sexual organs. In fact, the vulva can look very different from one girl to the next.

Interestingly, the vagina, which you have no doubt heard so much about, is not considered one of the external organs, but is part of the internal organs, explored later in this chapter.

At the very top of the woman's sexual organs is a mound of fatty tissue covering the pubic bone. This is called the **mons pubis**. The mons becomes covered with hair during puberty. This hair, which usually surrounds the vulva as well, is called **pubic hair**.

Below the mons are two folds of skin referred to as the outer lips, or **labia majora** (*lay*-bee-uh mu-*jor*-ruh) (Latin for "major lips"). Inside of these lips can be found another set of smaller lips, called **labia minora** (*lay*-bee-uh min-*nor*-uh) (Latin for "minor lips"). These inner lips are very sensitive during sex play.

At the top of the inner lips, where they come together, is located a small, pea-sized bit of flesh called the **clitoris** (*klit*-or-is). Although it looks like a tiny unimportant piece of tissue, the clitoris is the most sensitive part of the woman's sex organs. It is a place where many nerve endings come together, and for most women is the most sensitive part of their body. Just like the penis has two parts, the shaft and the glans (tip), so does the clitoris have a shaft and glans. In fact, the same spongy material that makes the penis get erect also helps the clitoris get somewhat erect when it is sexually stimulated.

Because the clitoris is so sensitive, many men believe that it is important to bring the penis in contact with the clitoris during intercourse. This is a myth! During intercourse, as the female partner approaches

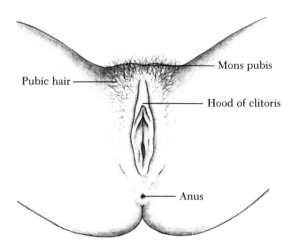

Pubic hair — Mons pubis

Hood of clitoris

Anus

(A) Vulva in normal state and

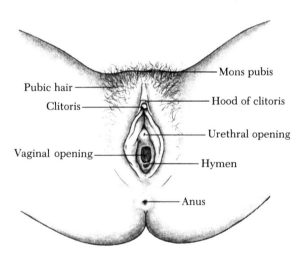

Pubic hair — Mons pubis

Clitoris — Hood of clitoris

Urethral opening

Vaginal opening — Hymen

Anus

(B) when stretched apart

Figure 10

orgasm, the clitoris goes behind a small piece of skin called the **clitoral hood.** As the penis goes in and out of the vagina it pulls slightly on the hood, which rubs against the sensitive clitoris. This is what causes so much of the pleasurable sensations for a woman during intercourse even though the penis at no time comes in direct contact with the clitoris. Often women enjoy stimulation of the clitoris manually (by hand) during foreplay or sometimes during intercourse.

Internal Organs

Inside the labia minora can be found two small openings. The opening on top, the urethra, is a short tube that connects to the bladder and is responsible for carrying urine for elimination from the body. The lower opening is the vagina.

The vagina is a short passageway, about four inches long, located between the urethra and the anus. The vagina is not a hollow space, as you might expect, but rather its sides touch each other. The walls of the vagina are wrinkled and, during sexual intercourse, the vagina actually widens and lengthens to adjust to the size of the penis.

When girls are born, the vagina is usually covered by a thin piece of tissue with one or more holes in it called a hymen (maidenhead). Although some cultures view the absence of a hymen in a maturing female as a sign that she has had intercourse at least one time and is thus no longer a virgin, this is not necessarily the case. Some girls are born without hymens, and many others have their hymens separated while participating in sports or other physical activities.

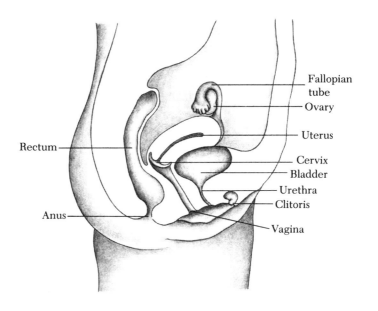

Figure 11 Female internal organs

If the hymen has not been previously separated, it is usually punctured during the girl's first experience with intercourse. This may result in a small amount of pain and slight bleeding. This bleeding may be the origin of the expression "she lost her cherry," which means that a girl experienced intercourse for the first time.

At the inner end of the vagina lies the **uterus**, or womb. This is a hollow organ with thick, muscular walls. It is the place where a baby is carried during pregnancy. The end of the uterus that connects with the vagina is known as the cervix. Before a woman becomes pregnant the uterus is about the size of an adult fist, but during pregnancy it adjusts to the size of the growing baby.

Leading into the uterus are the two **fallopian tubes**. Each of these carry eggs from the **ovaries** on a four-inch journey down to the uterus. The ovaries are two almond-shaped organs, each about an inch in length. From the day a girl is born, each ovary contains thousands of tiny eggs. Once she enters puberty, the eggs are released at a rate of approximately one per month. No eggs are released when a woman is pregnant. For most women, only three to five hundred of these eggs are released during their lifetimes. The ovaries are also responsible for the production of hormones that are instrumental in the growth and maturing process of girls and in the regulation of their menstrual cycles.

Understanding a Girl's "Periods"

Boys often make all sorts of jokes about girls having "**period**s" and about girls wearing sanitary napkins or tampons, but few boys understand this seemingly mysterious event that girls go through. The actual name for a period is **menstruation**, and for most girls it occurs about every twenty-eight to thirty days. Actually, menstruation is only one part of a whole series of events called the menstrual cycle, which goes on in a female's body every month.

The menstrual cycle starts when a single egg begins to mature inside of one ovary and gradually works its way through the surface of the organ. This process takes about two weeks. Finally, the mature egg breaks its way through the ovarian walls and into the fallopian tubes. This process is known as **ovulation**.

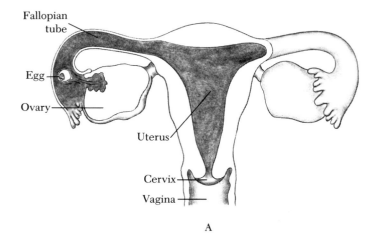

A

(A) Ovulation—an egg is released from the ovary into the fallopian tube. (B) The egg travels down the tube to the uterus. The uterine lining thickens and readies for the implantation of a fertilized egg. (C) If the egg does not implant, the lining of the uterus is shed. The blood and tissue leave the body through the vagina.

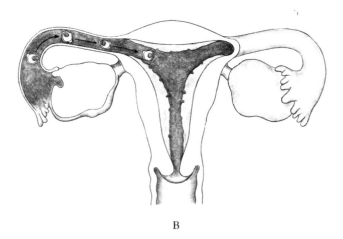

B

Figure 12 The process of menstruation

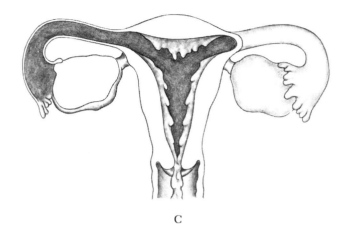

C

Gradually, the egg makes its way down the fallopian tube on a three- or four-day journey that carries it to the uterus. As this process is occurring, the walls of the uterus form a lining and grow thicker, preparing for the possibility of the woman becoming pregnant. If the woman does become pregnant, this lining will protect and nourish the fertilized egg.

If the egg is not penetrated by the male's sperm before the egg leaves the fallopian tube and enters the uterus, the woman does not become pregnant. The egg and the lining of the uterus then slough off and are expelled through the vagina with a small amount of blood. It is this mixture of tissue, blood, and some mucus leaving the body that is known as the menstrual period.

Because the hormones that regulate menstrual cycles are very sensitive to emotional and physical changes, for some girls the length of their menstrual cycles may be very unpredictable. For example, in situations when a girl is emotionally upset or loses a great deal of weight, her period may be delayed. This is one reason why the rhythm method of contraception is often unreliable. For some women the hormone changes that occur during the menstrual cycle may lead to changes in their mood during the month. For some women these mood changes are very severe, while for others these changes are hardly noticeable.

A female's periods occur about every twenty-eight to thirty days from the time she enters puberty until the time her ovaries stop producing female hormones. This time when the hormones cease usually occurs when the woman is in her late forties (although the age can vary) and is referred to as **menopause**.

Breasts

For a maturing boy, a girl's breasts seem to hold more fascination than any other part of her body. Many times it seems like a highly sexual game to try to take a peek down a girl's loose blouse or to accidentally on purpose brush your elbow or hand against her breast (we used to call this "copping a feel"). The thought of seeing or feeling even a portion of a breast can seem almost like a sexual experience in itself. Magazines such as *Playboy*, where women's breasts are readily visible, seem to take on the value of a treasure of gold.

However, along with the fantasy of breasts come the myths and exaggerations. Breasts are not all large and are not necessarily shaped like those of the women in *Playboy*. Breasts come in all sizes and shapes, but neither the size nor the shape has anything to do with how feminine a female is.

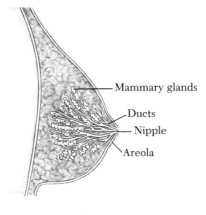

A

(A) Cross section of a female breast and **(B)** three various shapes of breast.

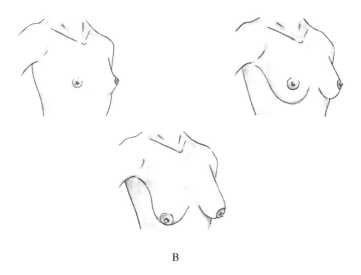

B

Figure 13

Although it is true that most females, as part of the process of sexual play, do enjoy having their breasts touched, other females get no pleasure at all from breast stimulation. In addition, if a girl is not in a sexual mood, touching her breast may be annoying to her.

A common myth among boys is that a girl's breasts are filled with milk. Actually the breasts are made up mostly of fatty tissue. There are glands in the breast that can produce milk, but unless a woman is in late pregnancy or is **nursing** a baby (feeding it her breast milk) after pregnancy, no milk is present.

Besides the fatty tissue, the breast contains the **mammary glands**, which produce milk when necessary, and ducts (passageways), along which the milk travels until it reaches the **nipple**. The nipple is at the tip of the breast. Nipples also come in all sizes and shapes. Some may stick straight out and others may turn inward. They tend to get more erect when a woman is cold or when she is sexually stimulated. When an infant feeds at the mother's breast, it squeezes the darker area around the nipple called the **areola** and sucks instinctively at the nipple, pulling the milk out of the ducts. The areola may vary in color from dark brown to pink, and sometimes has tiny bumps.

Although all females have the same basic parts to their bodies, it is important to remember that every body is different. Every girl's body looks somewhat dissimilar, and every girl's body responds differently to her menstrual cycle. Emotionally and sexually also, every female is unique. Just as you know that you are different from all other boys, each girl is an individual unlike any other girl.

12

SEXUAL DIFFERENCES AND PROBLEMS

I am sure that there are some times when you worry whether there is something wrong with you or if somehow you are different from your friends. All teenagers do. The truth is, *You are different.* You are different from anyone else. Just look in a mirror. Do you know anyone who looks exactly like you? Certainly you may have some features that resemble your parents or you may look similar to a brother or sister, but when you come right down to it, *you are unique.*

Sexually too you are unique. Your feelings, your beliefs, your thoughts, and your values are unlike anyone else's. Physically, your body looks and responds differently than other boys'. Even your penis is somewhat different in size and shape than most of your friends'.

How Different Am I?

If you want to find out if you are of average height, it certainly is easy enough. You use a yardstick, measure your height in inches, and then compare that with other boys your own age. The same goes for weight. You step on a scale, determine the number of pounds you weigh, and again compare yourself to other boys. Comparing height and weight are simple because there are standard units of measuring height and weight that our society has agreed upon. Everyone gets measured in inches or weighed in pounds. If two boys are sixty-five inches tall, we know that they are the same height.

When it comes to sex, however, there is no standard unit of measurement. We don't measure sex in inches, pounds, degrees, or any other unit of measurement. You can't measure that your sexuality is twenty-four and your friend's is twenty-one, so you are more sexual than he is. You can't decide if you feel okay sexually by comparing yourself to other people. If you are looking for a yardstick to measure yourself sexually, all you will find is confusion.

The following section includes a number of sexual differences that are often uncomfortable to teenage boys. Since some of these topics would be interesting mainly to someone who is experiencing these differences, you might find that you are not interested in all of them. In that case, simply scan the headings until you find one that might seem of interest to you. For the most part, these differences are part of the normal variety with which nature provides us. Some of the people who experience these differences do so comfortably or even proudly. However, others may feel uncomfortable, abnormal, or even ashamed. If one of these differences does cause you serious emotional upset, suggestions are included under each subsection to assist you in getting help. And the Appendix has more detailed information about help for these problems.

Differences in Sexual Feelings

Am I Too Sexual?

Just as there are some people who desire more or less food than others, there are people with greater or lesser sexual appetite. Actually, since much of your sexual cravings are regulated by hormones, you have little control over how sexual you feel. You are, in a sense, a victim of your own body.

If your body is constantly flooded with some of these chemical messengers, as a teenage boy's body often is, then it is likely that your sexual drive will be fairly strong. Most teenage boys, because of the action of these hormones, feel very sexual (horny) much of the time. Often sexual thoughts will occupy a good deal of their waking and even their sleeping hours. Sometimes the feeling can become so uncontrollable that the boy begins to feel that he has a serious sexual problem. These strong and sometimes overwhelming feelings are simply a need by the teenager's body to release a tremendous amount of sexual energy. The following is the case of a teenage boy who thought he was going crazy because he no longer understood his actions.

Robert was a friendly boy, well liked by his friends, family, and teachers. He was aware of his growing interest in girls from about the age of ten and, at about age fourteen, began to feel a greatly increased sexual desire. He was uncomfortable with the idea of masturbation and felt too shy to approach any girl with the idea of dating.

As the sexual urge grew inside of his body, Robert began to feel almost like two separate people. He knew he was still the quiet, well-liked boy that others had enjoyed, but he also felt so overwhelmed by the sexual urges that he began to feel crazy. One day, when calling for a friend of his who happened not to be at home, he began to talk with the friend's seventeen-year-old sister. As he chatted, he became aware of what felt like overwhelming sexual feelings just from talking with her and looking at her fully developed body. As the talking began gradually to change to teasing, the two of them began playfully to wrestle with each other. To his surprise, after a minute or so of wrestling, without any real sexual contact, Robert ejaculated just from having his body in close contact with hers. The sensation of "coming" felt tremendously good to him. However, along with the intense pleasure of the physical release of the orgasm, he felt guilt about having done something wrong, as well as a worried feeling that she would notice the wet spot on his pants or the smell of the semen.

After this incident, he went to his friend's house often, knowing his friend wasn't home. Each time he baited the sister into a wrestling match, and each time the result was the same—a feeling of tremendous sexual relief followed by embarrassment. In addition he felt fear that someone would discover what he was doing, and a feeling that he must be weird for repeating such bizarre behavior.

Robert's behavior, as he later found out, was not as strange as it seemed. He had found a way of releasing a tremendous amount of stored-up sexual energy in a way that was playful and pleasurable.

In some ways, feeling very sexual can be very pleasant. However, to many teenagers, all it means is a great deal of sexual frustration. Although some adolescents reduce this frustration either through masturbation or sex play with a partner, others find themselves trapped with feelings that they do not feel comfortable in expressing.

Being trapped with sexual feelings is like being in any other trap. It feels frustrating and often scary. If you find yourself in a position where those frustrations and scary feelings are becoming too overwhelming, it makes a big difference if you can share those feelings with a parent, or any adult you can trust. It may even be helpful to seek out counseling. A psychologist or counselor who works frequently with adolescents, or a counselor from one of the agencies listed in the Appendix, can often be of great help.

Am I Not Sexual Enough?

Not all males share Robert's problem. Many boys and men worry that they do not have enough sexual drive. After comparing themselves to all the exaggerations and lies of other males, and to the image of men that is portrayed by books and films, they become concerned that their sexual drive is not like that of other males.

The truth is that there is a tremendous range of sexual feelings in both men and women. Some men feel sexual much of the time, while others seldom feel sexual. As was indicated in chapter 7, "Your Penis Can

Talk," the fact that one person's sexual drive can be higher or lower than another's can be caused by many factors—physical, psychological, social, et cetera.

If you feel you do experience an unusually low sexual drive, it might be helpful to discuss your fears with a parent or other trusted adult. However, unless your concerns about not feeling sexual become very serious, or unless you know that you have gone through a serious problem in your life that has turned you off toward sex, professional counseling for this problem is not always immediately necessary. If, on the other hand, you find a partner to whom you feel really close, and you and your partner feel that your sex drive is still too low, counseling by a certified sex therapist would be appropriate. Likewise, if you are so averse to sex that you avoid getting close to possible partners, sex therapy would be indicated.

Differences in Sexual Identity

Homosexuality

One aspect of sexual differences that gets a great deal of attention among teenagers, yet is probably one of the least understood areas, is homosexuality. The terms "**gay**," "**fag**," or other slang synonyms are often thrown at other teenagers as a way of teasing, hurting, playing, or describing anyone who appears to be "different." A boy who is quiet and shy might be called "gay." A boy who is sensitive and cries or one who dresses unusually might be called a "fag." None of these have anything to do with homosexuality.

A **homosexual** is a person whose primary means of receiving sexual pleasure is with members of his own sex. A female homosexual is referred to as a **lesbian**. Someone whose primary means of receiving sexual pleasure is with the opposite sex is referred to as a **heterosexual**.

For many teenage boys, homosexuality is a confusing and scary topic. Rarely is homosexuality discussed between boys. If it is "talked about," it is almost always in the form of a joke or a negative remark. Consequently, a great deal of misinformation has developed on what homosexuality is all about. The following are some of the most common myths about homosexuality, followed by some facts to make it more understandable.

Myth 1: You can tell a homosexual by the way he acts, dresses, or talks.

Fact 1: For the most part, homosexuals do not look, dress, or talk differently than heterosexuals. Certainly there are some "gays" (this is a commonly used synonym for homosexual) who appear to act or dress strangely, but then again there are many "straights" (a commonly used synonym for heterosexual) who likewise act in a strange or unusual manner. Most homosexuals appear indistinguishable from heterosexuals.

Myth 2: Homosexuality is an indication that a person has some serious psychological problems.

Fact 2: Most psychologists, psychiatrists, and other mental health professionals now agree that homosexuality is not a mental disorder. Rather, they believe that homosexuals are simply people who have different sexual interests than heterosexuals. Many homosexuals lead a perfectly comfortable life and appear to have no more mental problems than do heterosexuals. Eleven percent of the men surveyed for *The Hite Report on Male Sexuality* reported that their sexual relations were primarily or exclusively homosexual, while an additional 4 percent of the men in that study reported enjoying sex with both men and women.

Myth 3: Any male who engages in any sexual activity with another male is a homosexual.

Fact 3: This is an extremely confusing point for many teenagers. Many boys engage in sex play with other boys during their growing years. This kind of harmless experimentation is common and normal among children and early adolescents. However, sometimes fear and a lack of understanding of homosexuality lead adolescents to unnecessary guilt and doubts about this type of experience.

Larry was eleven when out of curiosity he and a fifteen-year-old boy began to experiment sexually with each other. The experimentation only occurred twice, but Larry carried with him for years both the memories of the physical pleasure and a feeling of extreme guilt resulting from the belief that he had done something terribly wrong. Both the positive and the negative memories were extremely strong. Since this had been the one pleasant sexual experience in his life, he would sometimes fantasize about it as a way of "turning himself on" during masturbation. At other times when he masturbated, he fantasized about girls. Unfortunately, although he felt attracted to girls, his attempts to gain their attention always seemed to end with his getting teased or made fun of. Gradually, as he began to feel more unsuccessful with girls, his sexual fantasies about them began to decrease. To fill his need for fantasy during masturbation, he gradually increased his thoughts about the pleasurable experience with the other boy.

As he got older, Larry avoided all sexual contact with both men and women. He felt completely "turned off" by any thought of being sexually involved with a male, but had labeled himself as a "homosexual" because all of his sexual fantasies were now of male relationships. He did feel some attraction to women, but was fearful that they would discover his "homosexuality."

After entering therapy, it took nearly two years for Larry to undo the damage he had brought upon himself. His lack of understanding about the two brief sexual incidents when he was eleven years old, together with an ignorance about sexuality and homosexuality, resulted in many years of unnecessary doubts about himself.

Myth 4: Homosexuality is an all-or-nothing thing. Either you are entirely heterosexual or you are entirely homosexual.

Fact 4: Actually classifying people as gay or straight is like trying to categorize your friends as short or tall. Some of them are clearly short, and some are clearly tall, but some fit somewhere in between. Some men who are primarily heterosexual occasionally engage in homosexual acts, and some homosexual men engage sexually with women. In addition, there are some people who are referred to as **bisexual**, who enjoy maintaining sexual contact with both males and females.

Myth 5: Homosexuals are dangerous and are likely to force boys into engaging in sex with them.

Fact 5: Just by listening to the news or reading a newspaper, you hear about sex crimes against both children and adults. However, there is no indication that homosexuals are any more likely to commit these crimes than are heterosexuals. Unfortunately, we live in a society where sex crimes have increased over the past few years. However, children seem to be in no more danger from the gay community than from straights. It is true that many more sex crimes are committed by men than by women, but most of these are committed by heterosexual men against women. It is a good idea for all children and teenagers to stay away from any situations that will place them alone with any strange adult or even familiar adults who attempt to pressure them into sexual activity.

Most teenagers have occasional concerns about whether or not they have homosexual feelings. Yet, after they mature, they realize that their concerns were just a normal part of the confusion associated with growing up. On the other hand, some teenagers and adults go through tremendous fears about whether or not they are gay. Worries about homosexuality can be very upsetting. If this is a serious concern to you, talking about it would be worthwhile. If you feel that it would be impossible to talk to a parent or another close adult, seek help from a psychologist or other counselor.

Unfortunately, many parents and even many counselors and psychologists are not very comfortable in discussing homosexuality. If you do find someone to talk to, it is important that it is someone who is willing to explore both your homosexual and heterosexual feelings. If you find that the person with whom you are sharing your feelings seems to be strongly pushing you into becoming straight or gay, or, if you feel like he avoids the topic, it is likely that you need to find someone else to talk to. Choose someone who you feel can be open and honest with you.

Transsexuality

A condition that is often mistaken for homosexuality is transsexuality. **Transsexuals** are people who feel as if they are trapped inside a body of the wrong sex. Unlike a male homosexual who identifies himself as a male but prefers sex with other males, a male transsexual actually feels as if he is a female, trapped inside of the body of a male. Transsexuals can now be treated with a combination of surgery, hormones, and psychological counseling, so that they can appear and function as a member of the opposite sex.

Since very few professionals know much about dealing with transsexuals, it may be difficult to find a professional who can competently treat this problem. If you do have concerns about transsexuality, write to the J.T.C.P. (see page 211). They can refer you to a qualified professional.

Cross-Dressing

Cross-dressing is also often mistaken for homosexuality. **Cross-dressers**, or **transvestites** (as they are sometimes called), are people who feel some sexual satisfaction from dressing as someone of the opposite sex. Cross-dressers do not feel like they are actually members of the opposite sex, as do transsexuals, and most are not homosexuals.

Cross-dressing also should not be confused with the normal experimentation that children often go through, dressing up in their parents' clothes, or with the fun of dressing up as the opposite sex for a costume party.

At the present time, there does not seem to be any specialized type of treatment that is effective in dealing with people who cross-dress. If you do have concerns about cross-dressing, a psychologist or other counselor can be helpful.

Differences in Sexual Performance

Ejaculating Too Quickly

When a male and a female engage in a sexual relationship it is unusual for both partners to reach orgasm at the same time. Usually, males will tend to come somewhat before the female. With some males this orgasm is so quick their partners are left feeling frustrated because they too were not able to feel sexually satisfied. If the male, on a fairly consistent basis, quickly reaches the point of ejaculation but leaves his partner with only a sense of sexual frustration, the couple is likely having problems with **premature ejaculation**. This is the most common of all sexual difficulties reported by men.

It should be noted that it is not uncommon that sexual experiences with a new partner often result in quick ejaculations for many men. However, this is usually only considered to be a sexual problem if these premature ejaculations continue even after the relationship has continued for a while.

Premature ejaculation can often cause serious problems for a sexual relationship. However, of all sexual dysfunctions or problems, it is the most successfully treated. Premature ejaculation can be successfully reversed almost 100 percent of the time, with the help of a qualified sex therapist (see listing for AASECT under "Sex Education and Therapy" in the Appendix). On the other hand, home remedies, such as special creams or the use of prophylactics to lessen the amount of sensation, often have little success. Often, these remedies decrease the enjoyment of the sexual experience. Another often-used remedy by men who suffer from premature ejaculation is to think about things other than the sexual experience in an effort to cut down the degree of sexual excitement and thus help them control their ejaculations. Unfortunately, they too often find that this "cure" cuts down on their sexual pleasure and sometimes even leads to problems that are more diffcult to treat.

Not Ejaculating At All

A much rarer problem than premature ejaculation, but one that causes great concern among some men, is the inability to ejaculate at all during intercourse. Some of the men who experience this problem feel a sensation of orgasm but find that no semen spurts out of their penis, while others feel no orgasm at all. This lack of ejaculation does not occur frequently among teenagers.

This problem can be either psychological or physical in nature or may be the result of taking certain medications. The initial evaluation for this problem should be done by a physician, preferably a urologist. If the physical examination does not reveal any problems, then evaluation by a certified sex therapist would be the next step.

Impotence

Impotence is the inability of a male to get an erection sufficient to complete intercourse. Although all men face occasional difficulties in getting or maintaining an erection, some men fear these failures throughout almost all of their sexual experiences. For these men, impotence can lead to serious psychological problems if left untreated.

As indicated in chapter 7, there can be many reasons for a male's failure to get an erection. Consequently, treatment for impotence may be medical, psychological, or both. Psychologically based impotence can be reversed about 70 percent of the time, whereas the possibility of reversing impotence caused by medical reasons depends upon the medical cause. If these remedies are not successful it is now possible, with the help of surgery, for a device called a **prosthesis** to be placed inside the penis, which allows it to be inflated (similar to a long balloon) using a tiny pump.

Repeated experiences with impotence should be evaluated by a certified sex therapist and by a urologist with considerable experience in the area of male sexual problems. Any medications you are taking should be thoroughly evaluated by a physician to make sure that the impotence is not being brought on by side effects. This is especially true for medications used to control high blood pressure.

Not Satisfying My Partner

In some ways this is a problem that men worry about much too much. If your partner is not feeling sexually satisfied, there is a shared responsibility. First of all, it is her responsibility to share what her needs are. Secondly, it is your responsibility to listen to her needs. You don't necessarily have to do everything that your partner requests, but at least pay attention.

In addition, don't assume that your partner is not enjoying sex because she does not reach orgasm during each experience with intercourse. Although most men reach orgasm every time, most women do not. Certainly, women enjoy the orgasmic experience and prefer the same complete satisfaction and release that men do, but most women are not as "hung-up" about having orgasms as the men they are with. Women often enjoy sexual experiences without having an orgasm. Trying to push your partner into having an orgasm will likely cause her considerable pressure and often will result in her enjoying the sexual experience even less. Listen to your partner, don't push her.

Forced Sexual Encounters

Although most people seem to think about rape and forced sexual involvement (molestation) as a problem that females experience, it is likewise a serious problem for boys. Every year there are many thousands of situations in which boys are forced to perform sexually by strangers, relatives, friends, and even parents or stepparents.

Sometimes a man is able to pass off a molestation that occurred when he was an adolescent as simply a bad memory that he would rather forget. However, for many other men who have suffered the pain of having been molested, the emotional scars are very deep and painful. Some men suffer emotional problems their whole lives because they were the victims of such molestations. This is particularly true when the victim was repeatedly molested over a long period of time.

Karl was ten years old when his father divorced his alcoholic mother and twelve when his father remarried. His stepmother was good to him and his younger brother, but occasionally she would fly into an unexplained rage and would take it out on the boys. During these periods she would whip the boys, particularly the younger brother. During one of these episodes, while protecting his brother, Karl found that his stepmother became soothed when he put his arm around her and stroked her back. Her anger and rage seemed to disappear almost magically.

His stepmother began to encourage his stroking more and more, gradually leading his hands down to the area of her genitals. Eventually his stepmother encouraged him to engage in oral sex with her. Although Karl felt guilty and upset with this contact with his stepmother, he was relieved to have found a way to avoid the painful experience of being whipped or watching his brother being whipped. Because of this relief, and because he feared that his father would blame him for this sexual contact, he kept these incidents to himself. Through a combination of his own guilt and fear, and even some degree of sexual excitement, Karl continued this way of reducing his stepmother's tension until he decided to leave the house at age sixteen.

Karl's teenage and adult years were plagued with a great deal of sexual confusion. Karl married a number of times, each time feeling much guilt about sex. He tried to use sex as a way of reducing the tension at home when his wife was angry at him, but found that none of his wives responded by reducing their anger the way his stepmother did.

After years of therapy, Karl now understands the basis for many of his problems and is now settled in a stable marriage. However, he still finds it difficult to relate to women in any way other than sexually. For Karl it will take many years to undo the conflicts that his relationship with his stepmother caused in him.

Although the case is not typical, in that most boys who are molested are victims of other males, the fear and the guilt that Karl experienced are typical. Often it is difficult for the victim to decide whether to tell someone or not, particularly in cases where a parent or relative is involved. Unfortunately, this makes it impossible for either the victim or the child molester to get the help they so desperately need.

If you are ever the unfortunate victim of child molestation or know of someone who is, it is important that you share that information with an adult. If you feel you can, tell your parents. If you feel that they will not understand, contact an agency such as Family Service (see Appendix) or any other counseling agency. They will act to end the molestation and to get the victim the necessary help and support.

13

DEALING WITH
AN UNPLANNED
PREGNANCY

Whether or not your sexual partner becomes pregnant, this is an important chapter for you. It is important because it makes it clear that when you become
sexually active with a female partner, both of you take
some serious risks—not just your partner—*both of you.*

Boys tend to think of pregnancy as a problem that
girls face, and certainly in most cases it is the girl that
faces the most serious physical and emotional risks
from a pregnancy. However, boys also face serious
consequences, emotional and legal, which can affect
them for the rest of their lives. For example, if your
partner has a child as the result of your sexual activity
with her, you are legally the father of that child. This
means that a court of law can require you to contribute to the support of the child. This is a serious responsibility, which should not be taken lightly.

It is important to recognize that most "accidental"
pregnancies are not accidental at all. As the following
case illustrates, most teenage pregnancies occur either
because the couple lacked adequate knowledge about

birth control, or because they felt that pregnancy was something that happened to "other people."

Don and Tina were both seventeen when they began having intercourse. Although Don had picked up some information about using condoms from talking with other guys, he lacked any real knowledge about birth control techniques. Tina, on the other hand, had a fairly good knowledge about birth control pills, stemming from a talk she had with her mother when Tina was about fifteen. In that conversation, her mother had explained the importance about safe contraception and had told her where she could get birth control pills when she felt she needed them. Consequently, when Tina realized that she and Don were getting close to the point of engaging in intercourse, she went to her local Planned Parenthood clinic and obtained a prescription for birth control pills.

For one and a half years Tina continued to take the pill, and for that period of time she and Don continued to have intercourse with the assurance that she was protected from pregnancy. However, after being on the pill for such a long time, Tina gained about ten to fifteen pounds and started becoming concerned that she was looking unattractive. Realizing that weight gain is a frequent side effect of birth control pills, she decided to discontinue her use of the pill. She and Don talked about the situation, and agreed that a condom would provide them with the protection they needed. Not realizing that the use of a condom alone has a much higher failure rate than when used with spermicidal foam, they proceeded having intercourse with a false sense of confidence.

Within four months, Tina became pregnant: she was a victim not of an "accidental pregnancy" but rather of ignorance about birth control methods.

Pregnancy is not something that happens only to other people. It can very well happen to you. *There is no way absolutely to prevent a pregnancy.* As the accompanying table indicates, even if you and your partner use the best contraceptive methods available to teenagers, there is still a possibility of a pregnancy occurring. *If these contraceptive methods are not used correctly or if you use no contraception at all, the chances of your partner becoming pregnant are about nine out of ten over a one-year period of time.*

Contraceptive method	Percentage of pregnancies expected in all users (including those who use it carelessly and inconsistently) over a one-year period of time
No contraceptive used	90
Douche	40
Withdrawal	20–25
Rhythm (Calendar method)	21
Spermicidal foam	16
Diaphragm (using spermi- cidal foam or jelly)	10
Condom (alone)	10
Condom plus foam	5
IUD	5
Birth control pills	4

Even if you are lucky enough never to have to face the pain and anxiety of dealing with an accidental pregnancy, this chapter may still be helpful to you. From the latest statistics available, it can be estimated that over one million teenage girls will become pregnant this year. It is not unlikely that as you go through your high school years you will know a number of girls and boys who face the pain and anxiety of having to deal with an unplanned pregnancy. Possibly by reading through this chapter you will better understand the fear, anxiety, and confusion that these teenagers must experience, and, in addition, prevent yourself from getting into a similar predicament.

Is Your Partner Pregnant?

The first thing to do if your partner suspects that she is pregnant is to confirm whether or not she is. Some of the early signs that a girl will usually look for are a missed period (or sometimes only a shortened period), tenderness in the breasts, frequent urination, a feeling of nausea in the morning or late afternoon, or a feeling of being tired. However, even if a girl has missed a period and has some or all of the other symptoms, she still may not be pregnant. The only way a girl can be certain that she is pregnant is to have a laboratory test performed. This can be done either by a private physician or by an agency such as Planned Parenthood (listed in the Appendix). Even do-it-yourself pregnancy tests currently available at most drugstores cannot be relied upon. These home tests are fairly reliable only if used exactly as directed. However, because of a fear that parents may find the test, or for other reasons, many teenagers vary the directions slightly. This often fouls up the results. If your partner suspects that she is pregnant, confirm it with a test from a medical laboratory.

If She Is Pregnant

Possibly the two most feared words in the English language for the sexually active teenager are "I'm pregnant." If your partner tells you that she is pregnant, the two of you have some important decisions ahead of you. For most teenagers, this is an extremely frightening time.

After finding out that your partner is pregnant, it is likely that you will experience a period of intense emotions. Such emotions as fear, anger, sadness, anxiety, confusion, aloneness, and even pride may overwhelm your body. These emotions are very normal at a time when you face so many critical decisions.

The following is a discussion of some of the more important decisions that will have to be made.

Decision 1: Should I make any further decisions?
The first thing you must decide is how involved in the decision-making process you wish to become. You can either include yourself as a part of that process or you can dump all of the responsibility onto the girl. Remember, however, that many decisions will be made that will affect both of your lives. If you choose to pretend that this is the girl's problem and not yours, be aware that she will make the decisions—decisions that may seriously affect your life.

Ultimately, it is the girl who has the power to decide what the fate will be of the fetus growing in her body. However, you can be very helpful to her in making the monumental decision of whether she should carry the pregnancy to term (as opposed to having an abortion), and if so, whether or not she should keep the baby. In addition, you need to consider how important your relationship with this girl is to you. If you abandon her at this point, there is a good chance that the anger that will build in her will be enough to destroy your relationship.

If possible, try to become a part of the decision-making process.

Decision 2: How long can I postpone my decision?
When it comes to making critical decisions, many people seem to make either an instant decision, so they can remove the problem from their mind, or they try to postpone the decision in the hope that the problem will disappear. With an unplanned pregnancy, both of these are very poor ways of handling the problem.

There are too many important considerations with an unplanned pregnancy for you to make an instant decision. First consider all of the facts and feelings, and look carefully at each of the alternatives.

This is not a problem that will go away all by itself. It is not like waking up from a nightmare and feeling relieved when you realize that the scary dream is finally over. With a pregnancy, the decisions don't become any easier if you put them off. As a matter of fact, some of the alternatives, such as abortion (see the subsection about abortion later in this chapter), become riskier and sometimes impossible later in the pregnancy.

Take enough time to look carefully at all of the al-

ternatives, but do not avoid making the necessary decisions.

Decision 3: To whom can I go for guidance?

Another serious consideration for the two of you is whether you want outside guidance in looking at all the complicated aspects of this problem. Serious consideration should be given to sharing the problem with a trained counselor and with your parents.

Since everyone's situation is different, it is impossible to say that parents should always or should never be included in the discussions about resolving an unplanned pregnancy. This is a decision that you and your partner will have to make, based upon your own knowledge about your parents. If you choose to terminate the pregnancy with an abortion, this can often be done without your parents' knowledge and consent.

Whether or not you decide to include your parents, a trained professional counselor still can help you evaluate all of the complicated alternatives. If you have some doubts about telling your parents or the girl's parents, a counselor can help assist you in weighing all the advantages and disadvantages. Preferably, any counseling should involve both you and your partner.

You really have nothing to lose by going to a professional counselor, and possibly you might have a great deal to gain. Even if you disagree with what the counselor suggests, you still are free to carry out your own decision. Some of the agencies listed in the Appendix (such as Planned Parenthood) can provide you with such counseling or refer you to a qualified counselor.

Decision 4: What do we do about the pregnancy?

This is a very complicated decision. Basically, there are

three alternatives to consider. The first is for the pregnancy to be ended by means of an **abortion**. A second possibility is that after the child is born, one or both of the parents can raise the child. Marriage is often a consideration that goes with this second choice. The third alternative is for the pregnancy to continue and, after the birth, the child be given up for adoption or foster care.

As the following subsections of this chapter indicate, all of these alternatives involve some very complicated decisions. There are no easy answers.

Considering an Abortion

Abortion seems like an easy answer, and often is . . . for the boy. After all, as far as he is concerned, the girl goes to the clinic or hospital, checks in, goes through a brief medical procedure, and it's over . . . for him.

That is not what an abortion is all about. At least not from the girl's point of view. For most girls it is very scary to even think about going through an abortion, especially if she is planning on doing it without the knowledge of her parents. There may be fears about dying, of never again being able to have children, fears of killing an unborn child, or even religious pressures that bring about a feeling of guilt. These are very serious considerations for the girl, which the boy often does not face.

When performed by a trained professional, an abortion done in the first three months of pregnancy is usually a very safe medical procedure. The procedure generally takes from three to four hours, almost all of which is spent either taking tests or in recovery. The actual medical procedure takes only a few minutes.

During these early months of pregnancy, the most popular form of abortion is the vacuum-aspiration method. In this method, a small tube is inserted through the cervix, and the inside of the uterus is vacuumed out.

A second method, also used in early pregnancies, is referred to as a D and C (dilation and curettage). In this method, a small spoon is inserted and is used to scrape the walls of the uterus.

After the sixteenth week of pregnancy neither the aspiration method nor the D and C are used. Instead, the method of abortion most often used is the saline abortion. In this method, a salty solution is injected into the uterus. This solution kills the **fetus**, which is then ejected naturally from the body within about twenty-four hours, in a process similar to labor and delivery. This method of abortion can be very painful, both physically and emotionally, for a female. Whereas both the aspiration method and the D and C can usually be done in a clinic or office setting, the saline abortion requires that the girl be hospitalized for two or three days.

Although the courts have ruled that a minor does not need her parents' permission to have an abortion performed, many doctors require parental consent after the third month of pregnancy. This is particularly true when the saline method is used.

Abortions are legal throughout the United States up to the twenty-fourth week of pregnancy (although often it is difficult to find a doctor willing to do this procedure after twenty weeks). After the twenty-fourth week, abortions are legal only if the mother's life is endangered by the unborn child.

Abortions can sometimes create serious emotional pressures in women. Although women often heal quickly from the medical aspects of an abortion, often the emotional scars last much longer. Before, during, and after an abortion, a girl may need considerable emotional support from her partner and her friends. Be sensitive to that need.

Sometimes, in desperation, girls will even attempt to abort a pregnancy by themselves. Because they are afraid that their parents might find out, or because they are afraid they cannot afford the cost of a medically supervised abortion, many girls senselessly attempt home abortions, which can end up with their own death or disfigurement. Ironically, of course, in either case their parents do find out, and the financial and emotional cost to the family is considerably higher. Under any circumstances, do not allow your partner to try to abort the pregnancy by herself.

If abortion is the agreed-upon solution to a pregnancy, it should be done under the supervision of an experienced, qualified physician. To find out about the abortion facilities nearest to you, call one of the agencies listed in the Appendix, such as Planned Parenthood or Abortion Service.

Becoming a Father

A second alternative that many teenage couples who are faced with an unplanned pregnancy consider is having the child and becoming parents. However, like having an abortion, this alternative is not as simple as it may seem.

Certainly, having a child can be a wonderful experience for the couple that is prepared for it. However, for a young person unprepared for the responsibilities of parenthood a child can seem like a terrible burden. Children can be a lot of fun to play with or to baby-sit for. However, when the playing and the fun are over and you still have the responsibilities, being a parent is a lot of work.

Before you decide whether or not parenthood is the answer to a pregnancy, evaluate the following questions. Write down your answers, so that you can fully evaluate them when you are finished.

1. Can I earn enough to support a child?
2. How much time will I have to devote to work in order to support the child?
3. How much time will this leave me to give the child the amount of love and attention he or she will need?
4. How much time does that leave me to pursue the other plans for my future (school, career, personal plans)?
5. What plans for the future will I have to postpone or eliminate?
6. Can I be the kind of parent I would like to be?

Marriage

Another consideration that often goes with having a child is whether or not to get married. This is not the same as deciding whether or not to have the child. You do not have to get married just because a decision is made to have the baby. Certainly you will have some of the same responsibilities toward the child even if you don't have a marriage certificate. However, marriage is an additional responsibility on top of becoming a parent. If you decide to marry your pregnant partner, not only do you face the financial and emotional commitment to the child, but in addition, you are making a similar commitment to your partner.

If pregnancy is your only reason for getting married, then it is likely that the marriage will not be a very successful one. If, on the other hand, there are strong emotional ties between you and your partner, then the chances of a good marriage are somewhat better. In any case, be aware that the divorce rate for teenage marriages is extremely high. Marriage requires a great deal of work. It requires work to resolve arguments. It requires work to stay close when you are each under pressure. It requires constant work to figure out each other's responsibilities in the marriage. Love is not enough to make a marriage survive. There must be a commitment to constantly work and communicate in order to keep the relationship close. Before you make a decision to get married, make the same evaluation you did for having a child. Evaluate how much time you will need to devote to your wife and your marriage and how much this will alter your personal goals.

Having a child and getting married are two very different decisions. Before you decide on either, try to evaluate how the rest of your life might be affected.

Adoption and Foster Care

The third alternative is to give the baby up to be cared for by another couple. This can be done either through adoption or foster care. In adoption, the new couple permanently becomes the child's parents, and you no longer will have any legal rights as a parent. Foster care is a temporary situation, in which the child is given to the foster parents to care for until you or the mother is ready to permanently care for the child. Foster care should only be considered if you will be able to care for the child within a short period of time.

Giving a child up for adoption can be a very difficult sacrifice for a mother to make for her child. The maternal feelings that a mother has after giving birth to her child are often very strong. It is not unusual for a mother, after giving up her child to another set of parents, to go into a period of mourning, almost as if someone close to her had died. Like abortion, the alternatives of adoption and foster care tend to be much more painful decisions for women than they are for men.

A list of local or private agencies dealing in adoption and foster care can be obtained by contacting an agency such as the Florence Crittenton Association or Planned Parenthood (both listed in the Appendix).

14

A NEW ERA
IN SEXUALITY: AIDS,
SEXUAL RESPONSIBILITY
AND SAFE SEX

Without a doubt this is the most important chapter in this book. Your life and the lives of your sexual partners rest with your understanding of this chapter. As the title of this chapter indicates, this is truly a new era of sexuality. The spread of AIDS in our society has added a new and deadly dimension to our considerations about being sexually active. No longer is it possible to think about the pleasures of sexuality without considering the risks. Unless you understand what it means to be sexually responsible, and unless you realize that COMPLETELY SAFE SEX IS VIRTUALLY IMPOSSIBLE, you are unprepared to engage in any sexual activity with a partner. Read this chapter carefully and make sure you fully understand it.

AIDS (Acquired Immune Deficiency Syndrome)

AIDS is the newest and deadliest STD to reach public attention. Virtually unheard of before 1981, this disease has already claimed the lives of more than 24,000 people, with 42,000 more cases already reported in the U.S. Projections indicate that this may increase to between 220,000 to 400,000 cases by 1991. The disease is caused by the HTLV-III virus. However, because it slowly destroys the body's immune system, leaving it vulnerable to many illnesses, the name commonly used for the virus is HIV (Human Immunodeficiency Virus). Although technically it is incorrect to refer to it as the AIDS virus, since not all those with the virus have gotten AIDS, it will be referred to as both HIV and the AIDS virus in this chapter.

The seriousness of AIDS, and the publicity it has generated, has led to some myths and misconceptions about how one gets it, who is at risk, and how to prevent the disease. The following pages hopefully will dispel these myths for you and give you some accurate information. However, our knowledge of AIDS is changing every day. Realize that it is your responsibility to keep up to date on the current information. You can do this only by reading newspapers or calling one of the several AIDS agencies listed in the appendix. Do not trust the information given to you by friends without checking it out yourself. And because of the seriousness of this disease, if you are going to make an error in judgment, make it in the direction of being overly cautious rather than not cautious enough.

Who Can Get AIDS

Although much of the early publicity about AIDS indicated that it was male homosexuals, intravenous drug users, hemophiliacs, and Haitians who were particularly vulnerable to this disease, more recent statistics are indicating that the disease can be spread through heterosexual intercourse as well. Teenagers often have a way of minimizing the potential risk of their actions. Do not make the possibly fatal mistake of underestimating the risk of getting AIDS if you do not act in a sexually reponsible manner.

Some projections are indicating that one of the most at-risk groups for AIDS over the next few years may be teenagers, both male and female, heterosexual and homosexual. In fact, one recent report indicates that for the first 5 months of 1987, the number of AIDS cases among persons 13 to 19 years nearly doubled over the number for the same period in 1986, and nearly tripled the 1985 statistics for a like time period.

How is AIDS Spread?

AIDS is spread only when the fluids from an infected person are introduced into the body of another person. In people who are infected, the AIDS virus has been found in virtually every one of their body fluids. However, because just the right environment is necessary for the AIDS virus to survive outside the human body, and because it is believed that a healthy body probably can fight off the small amounts of virus found in infected saliva or tears, the disease is primarily spread either through intimate sexual contact or through contact with infected blood. Casual kissing does not appear to spread AIDS. However, because saliva and sometimes blood (from gum bleeding) are exchanged in deep kissing (French kissing, wet kissing), scientists have not ruled out that the virus, under certain conditions, might be transmitted in this manner.

Sexual Contact

The most common way in which AIDS is spread is through sexual contact. Whether you are heterosexual and homosexual, male or female, black or white, you are at risk if you engage in vaginal intercourse, anal intercourse, oral sex, or any other type of sexual activity in which a bodily fluid is discharged. It is believed that semen is responsible for spreading approximately two-thirds of the cases of AIDS. It should be noted, however, that withdrawal of the penis before ejaculation is not sufficient to stop the spread of AIDS. Evidence indicates that the fluids discharged from the penis prior to ejaculation also contain the virus. Anal intercourse is thought to be especially dangerous in spreading AIDS.

In addition, it has been shown that in infected women the virus is present in vaginal and cervical fluids during every stage of the menstrual cycle. Therefore, AIDS can be spread from females to males any time during the month. There is no safe time of the month when it comes to the transmission of AIDS.

Blood Transmission

Although there has been much publicity about individuals who have contracted AIDS from blood transfusions, this method of acquiring the virus accounts for only 2% to 3% of active cases. Methods of screening blood supplies have vastly improved, so there is now very little risk of contracting AIDS through this means. A far more common method of blood transmission is through the use of contaminated needles when sharing street drugs.

AIDS can also be spread to babies, either through the blood flow from an infected mother to her fetus prior to delivery, or from the mother's milk after delivery. The chance of an unborn child getting AIDS from her infected mother exceeds 50 percent.

Although the AIDS virus has also been detected in urine, stool, and other bodily fluids, there are no documented cases of transmission through these fluids.

Ease of Transmission

Because the AIDS virus is a fragile organism, it is not easily transmitted except through bodily fluids. The organism cannot live long outside the human body, and even then is easily killed by heat, alcohol, and diluted bleach. However, once the virus becomes entrenched in the human body, it is impossible to kill.

It also appears that the more repeated exposures to a virus a person has, the more likely he is to contract the disease. It has been shown that many sexual encounters with different partners or many exposures with one infected partner will increase the risk of contracting the AIDS virus.

Myths About the Spread of AIDS

It is clear that AIDS is not transmitted through casual contact with infected persons. There are no documented cases of friends or relatives, even those living with infected AIDS victims, getting the disease through casual contact. This includes hugging, casual kissing, or sharing food, kitchen utensils, bathroom facilities and other household facilities. Even children who play daily with infected friends have shown no signs of contracting the disease.

Another myth is that AIDS is strictly a gay disease. This is definitely not true. Heterosexuals as well as homosexuals get AIDS. However, there seem to be mixed reports as to the ease of transmission of AIDS during sexual contact between males and females. Some studies indicate that the virus can be readily transmitted during heterosexual contact while others indicate that there is far less danger in heterosexual contact than homosexual contact. Because the research is unclear at this time, you must take maximum precautions during every sexual encounter.

Tests have also been conducted to evaluate whether AIDS could be spread by mosquitoes. As of this time there is no evidence to indicate that this is a viable method of transmission.

Stages of Infection and Symptoms

Acute Infection and Asymptomatic Infections

A small number of people who become infected with the AIDS virus experience typical flu-like symptoms approximately 3 to 4 days after becoming infected. The symptoms may include fever, a feeling of tiredness, headache, and swollen glands, and may be accompanied by a peeling skin rash. However, most infected people show neither these nor any other visible symptoms. Rather, they enter directly into an asymptomatic or silent stage of the infection. During this stage they may be somewhat more susceptible to infections and other diseases, but otherwise show no severe symptoms. Even though they may be asymptomatic during this stage, they are very capable of passing the disease on to others. It is unclear how long this silent stage may last. It appears that within a 5-year period of time, at least 30% of those in this stage will develop symptoms and progress to the final two stages. There is some evidence that the asymptomatic stage can last as long as 15 years but that eventually all of those in this stage of the illness will eventually progress to the later stages.

ARC (Aids Related Complex)

Aids Related Complex (ARC) is a more advanced stage of the disease. It is during the ARC stage that others around the victim often first become aware of his illness. During this stage the symptoms include a persistent fever, night sweats, fatigue, unexplained and persistent weight loss, a peeling skin rash, diarrhea, and swelling of the lymph glands, especially those in the armpits, the back of the neck, and the rear of the mouth. The ARC stage can last from a few months to a number of years before progressing to what we refer to as AIDS.

AIDS

AIDS is the final stage of this cycle, and results when the immune system is so weak that it can no longer protect the individual against disease. The symptoms of AIDS depend upon what illnesses the person develops due to his disabled immune system. In addition to all the symptoms of ARC, the person sometimes develops a severe and potentially lethal form of pneumonia (pneumocystis corinii) a rare and deadly form of cancer (Karposi's sarcoma), tuberculosis, herpes, yeast infections, and many other severe illnesses. In some victims, the virus enters the brain and can lead to strange behavior, as well as deterioration of judgment and memory.

Ninety percent of those that enter this final stage die within 2 years.

Tests

Should I Be Tested For AIDS?

If you have engaged in any sexual behavior that puts you at risk for AIDS, the answer is an emphatic YES. The riskier your behavior and the more numerous your sexual contacts, the more often you should be tested. The benefits of being tested far outweigh any fears you may have. If you test HIV negative (meaning you don't have the AIDS virus), the test will no doubt relieve any anxiety you might have. If it is confirmed by testing that you do have the virus, this will enable you to start treatment earlier and allow you to take steps to protect yourself against running down your immune system. In addition it will alert you so that you take the necessary precautions to protect others and to warn those whom you think you may potentially have infected in the past.

If you answer yes to any of the following questions, you should definitely be tested for AIDS:

1. I have had intercourse with a person without using a condom, and I am not absolutely positive that that person has not had sexual contacts with any other person since 1979.

2. I am sexually active with a number of partners (even if you use condoms).

3. I have had sexual contact with a prostitute or other sexually promiscuous person since 1979 (even if you used a condom).

4. I am a male and have had sexual contact with another male since 1979.

5. I have had sexual contact with an intravenous drug user since 1979 (even if you used a condom).

6. I have used intravenous drugs and have shared a needle since 1979.

7. I am a female and have, since 1979, had sex with a male that I know or suspect of being bisexual (even if he used a condom).

8. I have, since 1979, had sex with someone from Haiti, Africa, or others areas of the world where AIDS is rampant (even if you used a condom).

9. I received a transfusion of blood or clotting factors between 1978 and 1985.

10. I had sexual contact with anyone whom I know to have received a transfusion between 1978 and 1985 (unless they have since tested negative for AIDS).

11. I am concerned that I may have come into contact with the AIDS virus.

12. I am a health worker and come into contact with the bodily fluids of others.

Where and When Do I Get Tested?

AIDS testing is now easily available. Remember, however, that the primary test used at this time, the ELISA (Enzyme-Linked Immunosorbent Assay) test, is not valid until 6 weeks to 1 year after you initially become infected. You can have it done through doctors' offices, hospitals, public health departments, public laboratories, free clinics, and at special AIDS testing centers set up in larger cities. Private laboratories will probably want a referral from a physician before they will test you. Also, some laboratories are now testing for AIDS by mail order. Preferably, deal with a physician or a laboratory you are familiar with, or at least ask a health professional whom you trust to refer you to a reputable lab. Because different test kits have different levels of accuracy, only deal with a testing facility where they have personnel who will explain to you what a positive test means, how to follow up on a positive test, and where counseling is available if your test is positive.

Going to your physician makes the results of your AIDS test part of your medical records, and therefore available under certain circumstances to insurance companies, public health officials, or to a court if subpoenaed for a lawsuit. Consequently, some laboratories now offer anonymous testing, in which you are identified only by a number. Another reason that anonymous tests have been so popular is the fear that if the knowledge leaks out that someone has tested positive, it might jeopardize that person's schooling, job, or insurability for health or life insurance. With anonymous testing, you call the laboratory by phone, identify your number, and the technician gives you your results.

Do not ever go to a blood bank just to have your blood tested. On rare occasions the test will read negative even in an infected person. In a blood bank, this blood will be used for transfusions and will most likely infect others.

The cost of AIDS testing varies widely, from a low of $20 to as much as $150. This usually includes re-testing that will be necessary if your test is positive.

What if your AIDS Test is Negative?

In most cases, a negative ELISA test indicates that you have not developed antibodies against the AIDS virus, and therefore you are not infected. However, be aware that "false negatives" do occur, although rarely. Also since the ELISA is an antibody test and will not detect the infection for anywhere from 6 weeks to 1 year after it occurs, the results indicate only that you were not infected 1 year ago. Any HIV infection that occurred after that might not test positive.

If your test is negative and you are sexually active with a number of different partners, or if you have a sexual partner who is active with others, it is recom-mended that you be tested at least twice each year.

What if My ELISA is Positive?

If your ELISA is positive, don't panic. It does not definitely mean that you are infected. Approximately

2 out of every 1000 ELISA tests given result in a "false positive." If the ELISA is positive, it should be repeated. If the second test indicates a positive result, then a Western Blot test should be performed to confirm that you have been infected with the AIDS virus.

If you have been confirmed as HIV positive, the first thing you should do is to get counseling and medical advice. Find out what a confirmed test means. Get all of your questions answered, and get the benefit of talking with a counselor who has worked with those who have tested positive. Although you are certainly at risk for developing ARC and AIDS, this is not necessarily the case.

However, take into consideration that not everyone will be able to deal effectively with this information. Discuss with the counselor who you should tell of your test results, and who you should not tell. An HIV infection is not something that you should deal with alone. You will need a great deal of support now and in the future.

Find a physician who works with a large number of HIV positive patients. He is likely to be the most up to date on new research and the intricacies of treatment. Also, do not deal with a physician who seems as if he is afraid to treat you. Go to someone who is comfortable with dealing with the HIV-infected patient.

Do not have sexual contact with anyone without first informing the person that you are infected. Even if you take every reasonable precaution, she is still at serious risk. If the person wants to make the decision to have sex with you, that is her decision, but even then, it is not recommended, and she should do it only after carefully evaluating and understanding the risks. Likewise, do not expose anyone to any of your bodily fluids.

Notify every sexual partner you have had subsequent to the earliest date you feel you could have been infected. They should have themselves checked for the HIV antibodies.

Do not donate blood. Besides being unethical to expose anyone to such a danger as receiving infected blood, it is illegal in most states. You may even be charged with attempted murder.

Let your doctors, dentists, and anyone else who may be exposed to your bodily fluids know that you are HIV-positive. This will allow them to take the appropriate precautions so that neither they, their staff, nor other patients are put in any risk.

If you are an intravenous drug user, be especially careful not to share your needles with anyone, no matter how thoroughly you sterilize them.

Do not have unprotected sexual contact with anyone else who is HIV-positive. Indications are that the more contact you have with the virus, the more likely it is that the disease will progress.

Treatment

There is presently no cure for AIDS or the HIV virus, although a number of pharmaceutical companies have been testing various anti-viral agents. One such drug, AZT, has been released for use by people with AIDS, and has shown promising results in slowing down the disease process in some victims. However, research scientists still seem to be a number of years away from finding a cure or an effective way of preventing one from getting the infection.

Sexual Responsibility & Safer Sex

Sex Can Still Be Fun

All this talk about AIDS and the serious risks connected with it probably is somewhat scary, and it should be. It's smart to be scared of something that can be seriously harmful to you. But that doesn't mean that it has to ruin the enjoyment of a sexual experience. Sex can be extremely pleasurable, but only if you take the worry out of it.

It's like having the chance to attend a party the night before your math final. You are sure it's going to be a great party, but you are also aware that if you go, there is going to be a price to pay. You anticipate that it's likely to be somewhat difficult to enjoy the party worrying about whether you understand your math well enough to do well on the exam, or being concerned that your parents might find out that you were out playing when you should have been home studying. Then, you first have to wait a week to get your grade, praying that you passed the class. There is no way that the party will be as enjoyable knowing the price you will have to pay.

With sexual responsibility the choices are similar, but the risks are far more serious. If you do not act in a sexually responsible manner it is going to be difficult to fully enjoy a sexual experience with the thought of AIDS in the back of your mind. Even if you can dismiss that thought temporarily and experience an hour of sexual ecstasy, you then have to worry for the next month whether your girlfriend is pregnant, or for the next year whether you have contracted AIDS or another STD. On the other hand, if you understand what precautionary measures are available to you, and use every one of them, your risks become extremely slight and your relaxation and enjoyment can grow tremendously. Sex can still be a great experience, but only if you fully understand how to protect yourself against any potential risks.

Deciding Whether or Not to Have Sex

The first decision you have to make is whether or not you feel that you want to be sexually intimate with a partner. For most teenagers, considering whether or not to have sex used to be a moral issue. Some felt that sex was not appropriate until after marriage or at least until they were in love. Now, there is an additional consideration. Abstaining from sex can be a safety issue—a way of protecting yourself and maybe even of preserving your life.

However, whether you decide to abstain or not, make sure your decision is a realistic one. Even if you decide to abstain, know how to protect yourself sexually. Don't make a decision to abstain and then find yourself in a passionate situation with a girl and no way of protecting yourself.

Understand that if you decide to engage in sexual intercourse or other intimate sexual contact you are taking on a serious responsibility. Not only are you responsible for your own health, but also for the health and welfare of your partner. If you do not know how to protect the two of you, and are not prepared to take all of those steps necessary, you are not prepared to be sexually intimate. Below are some of the measures that must be taken so that you can meet these serious responsibilities.

Safer Sex

You will notice that the name of this portion of the chapter refers to "safer sex," not "safe sex." That is because FOR MOST TEENAGERS, ABSOLUTELY SAFE SEX IS VIRTUALLY IMPOSSIBLE. This is not a "put down" of teenagers, it is simply a reality.

There is only one circumstance under which you can have absolutely safe sex, and that is with an absolutely safe partner. This means one that does not have the HIV virus, any other sexually transmitted diseases, and who cannot get pregnant. If you are going to be absolutely safe, you need to know that your partner has not had sex with anyone since 1979, has not had a blood transfusion since that date, has never used intravenous drugs, and has never been exposed to the bodily fluids of a person carrying the AIDS virus. Even if you asked all of the necessary questions, you would have to be absolutely sure that your partner was telling the truth.

Deciding Whether Your Partner is Safe

The first consideration about safety is KNOW YOUR PARTNER. Because it takes a lot of information to evaluate whether a partner is "safe," it is important to choose a partner whom you know well and whom you can trust. If you do not know much about your partner or are not sure whether or not she is trustworthy, then all of the information you need to evaluate her safety must be considered suspect.

Obviously, do not have sexual contact with anyone whom you know has tested positive for the AIDS virus. There is no way to absolutely protect yourself with someone who is HIV positive.

Ask your partner about her sexual history. Even if you feel it might be painful to know your girlfriend's sexual history, it is essential that you ask. The more lovers your sexual partner has had, the more risk there is that she has contracted the HIV virus. Even if she has slept with only one other person, if that person was sexually promiscuous, your chances of contracting the AIDS virus are greatly increased.

Also, having sex with anyone from one of the major at-risk categories greatly increases your chances of getting AIDS. Included in these categories are partners who are homosexual or bisexual, who have used intravenous drugs or have had health problems that might have required transfusions, or who are from Haiti or Africa. All of these partners are in a very high-risk group.

If you do have a situation where you have to make a difficult decision whether or not to be sexually intimate with a person from one of these high-risk groups, think strongly about not doing it. Consider the possible risk to your life, and evaluate all of the information in this chapter before making your decision. If you decide to take this serious risk, do so only after taking every precaution listed below.

How to Have Safer Sex

No matter how safe you believe your partner to be, never have sex without taking every precaution available. Remember, the risk that you face for believing the innocent voice of your partner is the possible loss of your life.

There are a number of things that you can do to lessen your chance of getting (or giving) AIDS. Since taking all of these precautions will also lessen the risk of pregnancy and of contracting most other sexually transmitted diseases, I will write only about avoiding AIDS.

Never have sex without using a latex condom, preferably one that is manufactured to include a contraceptive foam containing at least 5% nonoxynol-9. Latex condoms create a barrier so that the HIV virus can neither get in or out. Also, early tests indicate that nonoxynol-9, in addition to being an excellent spermicide, may be helpful in killing any of the AIDS virus that may be present.

Follow the directions in Chapter 5 about how to use a condom, being especially sure to withdraw immediately after ejaculation, holding the top of the condom. Immediately, throw the condom away, towel yourself dry, and do not make any contact again without using a fresh condom. Please note that animal-membrane condoms are not thought to be as effective as latex ones in preventing the spread of the HIV virus. Absolutely do not use any lubricants such as baby oil, cooking oil or salad oil, petroleum jelly (Vaseline), or any others that have any type of an oil base.

These will make latex condoms deteriorate and can lead to leakage.

Because condoms are not a foolproof means of preventing pregnancy, they likewise are not a perfect means of preventing the spread of AIDS. Consequently, in addition to using a condom, make sure that your partner is also using a foam that has nonoxynol-9. As with preventing conception, the combination of a condom and foam is much more effective than either method by itself. DO NOT place any foam inside the condom, as this will cause the condom to slip off.

As mentioned previously in this book (page 143), there are a great variety of sexual positions, some of which have special risks connected with them. Another aspect of how to have sex safely involves understanding what these special risks are and how to prevent them. Anal sex without a condom should be avoided. This is a position in which the penis is placed into the partner's anus. It is a position which is commonly preferred by homosexual males. Because it often results in some tearing of rectal tissues, and therefore some bleeding, this position is seen as highly risky in spreading AIDS.

Also, oral sex, either where the penis is placed into the partner's mouth or where the mouth is placed on the vagina, is likewise considered highly risky unless precautions are taken. These precautions include the use of a condom during oral sex to prevent any possible AIDS transmission from the semen, and use of a square of latex or plastic wrap (called an "oral dam") during oral stimulation of the female partner in order to prevent transmission through vaginal fluids.

If you are intending to be sexually intimate with a

partner, you owe it to yourself and your partner to take every precaution available. Do not take this risk lightly. The price of underestimating may be your life.

When to Have Sex

The final element of safe sex is when to make your decision. Never make a decision to have sex after having used drugs or alcohol. As with driving under the influence, your decision-making process becomes seriously impaired; and you are much more likely to make impulsive, unsafe decisions. If you are going to decide to be sexually intimate, do it while you are sober. At least then you are likely to look at the alternatives more reasonably and to take every precaution.

APPENDIX: FINDING HELP

We all need help now and then. None of us is completely self-sufficient. Yet asking for help can sometimes be a difficult thing to do. Even admitting that things are serious enough to require help may be difficult.

If you do find yourself in a situation that requires professional advice or assistance, competent help is usually available if you know how to find it. The following section is designed to ease the problems often connected with finding the proper professional help. It is divided into two parts.

1. How to find a referral in the telephone book.

2. A listing of various national agencies that you can write or call (many of them have toll-free numbers) to get information, or the name of a source of help close to your home.

Using the Phone Book to Find Help

Probably the easiest way to find help is to look in the white pages of your local phone directory under the word that best describes the service you require. For example, if you are looking for information about pregnancy, look in the white pages under the word *pregnancy*. If you are looking for birth control information, then look under *birth control* or even under *sex*. If you don't find the referral source that you need, look up *Planned Parenthood* or *Family Service*. Both of these are large national organizations with chapters in many towns and cities. Even if these organizations do not offer the type of service you need, it is likely that they can refer you to a place where you can get appropriate help.

A second way to use the phone book is to look in the yellow pages. The following are a partial list of headings that you might look under in searching for help.

Birth Control Information
Churches
Clergy
Clinics
Counseling
Crisis Intervention Services
Family Planning
Marriage Counselors
Mental Health Services
Psychiatrists
Psychologists
Social Service Organizations

Some yellow pages even offer an index in the back, where you can look up the specific service you want. Remember, if you call any organization and they do not offer the service that you require, ask them for suggestions as to where you might locate the kind of service you need. Many helping agencies are very aware of what resources may be available in your vicinity.

Organizations

The following is a list of national organizations that might be helpful in answering any questions you might have or in referring you to an agency in your vicinity that can be of assistance.

Abortion

National Abortion Hot Line
(800) 772-9100
Toll-free counseling, referral, and information services.

Florence Crittenton Association
440 1st St. N.W., Washington, DC 10003
(202) 638-2952
A counseling and referral organization with many affiliates, which explores alternatives to abortion.

Counseling and Referrals

Planned Parenthood Federation of America, Inc.
810 Seventh Avenue, New York, N.Y. 10019
(212) 541-7800
Offers medical, educational, counseling, and referral services for many aspects of sexuality, including the areas of birth control and sexually transmitted diseases. Has hundreds of affiliates throughout the country.

Family Service Association
254 W. 31 St., NY 10001
(800) 424-6268 or (800) 535-3222 (in New York)
A general counseling service with affiliated agencies throughout the United States.

Gay Services

Gay Switchboard
(215) 978-5700
A Philadelphia-based hotline providing information and referral services.

Gay Community Services Center
1213 North Highland, Hollywood, CA 90028
(213) 464-7400

National AIDS Hotline
(800) 342-2437
A toll free national hotline provided by the Public Health Service, which provides recorded information and additional phone numbers for people wanting referral or more information about AIDS.

Hotlines

Community Sex Information, Inc.
(212) 982-0052
A New York City-based hotline that provides information and referrals.

Sex Information Hotline
(213) 653-1123
A Los Angeles-based hotline that provides information and referrals.

Sex Education and Therapy

American Association of Sex Educators, Counselors, and Therapists (AASECT)
5010 Wisconsin Avenue NW, Suite 304, Washington, D.C. 20007
(202) 296-7205
A national professional organization of sex therapists and sex educators with members throughout the United States.

Sexually Transmitted Diseases

VD National Hotline (toll-free number)
(800) 227-8922
A toll-free counseling and referral service.

Transsexuality

J.T.C.P.

P.O. Box 184, San Juan Capistrano, CA 92693

(714) 496-5227

An information and referral source for those seeking information about transsexuality.

Recommended Readings

The following is a list of books and readings that might be useful for expanding upon the information presented in this book. For a child or a parent looking for quality reading material about sex, the array of books available can seem very confusing. The books are listed according to the topic areas they supplement.

Abortion

Corsaro, Maria, and Carole Korzeniowsky. *A Woman's Guide to Safe Abortion.* New York: Holt, Rinehart and Winston, 1983.

A realistic approach to the planning of an abortion. Also includes information on how to avoid future unwanted pregnancies.

Becoming a Young Parent

Gordon, Sol, and Mina Wollin. *Parenting: A Guide for Young People.* New York: William H. Sadlier, Inc., 1975.

Written for the young person preparing to become a parent.

Fiction

Blume, Judy. *Forever.* Scarsdale, N.Y.: Bradbury Press, 1975.
A novel written for teenagers, which gives a realistic view of teenage sexuality.

Homosexuality

Fairchild, Betty, and Nancy Hayward. *Now That You Know: What Every Parent Should Know About Homosexuality.* New York: Harcourt Brace Jovanovich, 1979.
A book helpful for parents trying to understand their homosexual child.

Hanckel, Frances, and John Cunningham. *A Way of Love, A Way of Life: A Young Person's Introduction to What It Means to Be Gay.* New York: Lothrop, Lee and Shepard (William Morrow), 1979.
A sensitively written book for the teenager trying to understand what it means to be gay.

More about Females

Eagan, Andrea Boroff. *Why Am I So Miserable If These Are the Best Years of My Life?* New York: Avon Books, 1979.
An understanding and factual account of the process of becoming a sexually mature young woman.

Voss, Jacqueline and Jay Gale. *A Young Woman's Guide to Sex.* Los Angeles: The Body Press, 1988.
A sex-education guide for the teenage girl that discusses realistically a young women's sexual and social concerns.

Wagenvoord, James, and Peyton Bailey, eds. *Women: A Book for Men.* New York: Avon Books, 1979.
A helpful book for men trying to broaden their understanding of women.

More about Males

Hite, Shere. *The Hite Report on Male Sexuality*. New York: Alfred A. Knopf, 1981.
   Results of a survey of over seven thousand men, listing and discussing some of the common (and uncommon) fears and sexual preferences of males.

Zilbergeld, Bernie. *Male Sexuality*. Boston: Little, Brown, 1978.
   A well-written, easily readable book for the man or woman trying to gain a more complete understanding of the physiology and emotional side of male sexuality.

Reproduction

Demarest, Robert J., and John J. Sciarra. *Conception, Birth and Contraception: A Visual Presentation*. New York: McGraw-Hill, 1976.
   A well-illustrated book for the middle-to-later teen about the process of human reproduction.

Sex for Teens

Hass, Aaron, Ph.D. *Teenage Sexuality*. New York: Pinnacle Books, 1981.
   Results of a survey in which teenagers discuss their attitudes about and expectations of sex.

Sex for the Disabled

Mooney, Thomas O., Theodore M. Cole, and Richard A. Chilgren. *Sexual Options for Paraplegics and Quadriplegics*. Boston: Little, Brown, 1975.
   An excellent source for helping the disabled person reach his or her maximum sexual potential.

Kempton, Winifred, Medora Bass, and Sol Gordon. *Love, Sex and Birth Control for Mentally Retarded: A Guide for Parents.* Planned Parenthood of Southeastern Pennsylvania, 1973.

A guide for parents of mentally handicapped children or adults about educating their child sexually.

Sexually Transmitted Diseases

Corsaro, Maria, and Carole Korzeniowsky. *STD: A Common-sense Guide to Sexually Transmitted Diseases.* New York: Holt, Rinehart and Winston, 1982.

A nonjudgmental, straightforward book for those interested in recognizing and understanding sexually transmitted diseases.

Gordon, Sol. *Facts about VD for Today's Youth.* Rev. ed. Fayetteville, N.Y.: Ed-U Press, 1979.

Information about sexually transmitted diseases; stresses the importance of prevention and early treatment.

GLOSSARY

AIDS—(Acquired Immunodeficiency Syndrome)—A deadly disease caused by the HIV virus. AIDS slowly destroys the immune system in the body and inevitably causes death.

Abortion—The ending of a pregnancy prematurely. The egg, the embryo, or the fetus (depending upon the stage of pregnancy) is removed or expelled from the uterus.

Acne—Large, deep pimples, which are common during adolescence.

Adolescence—The period of time beginning with puberty and ending with adulthood.

Anal sex (anal intercourse)—A form of sexual intercourse in which the penis is inserted into the partner's anus.

Androgen—A hormone that causes the male sex characteristics. Both males and females have androgens, although males have considerably more.

Anus—The opening of the body leading from the rectum, from which bowel movements are expelled from the body.

Aphrodisiac—Any substance that is thought to enhance sexual desire.

Areola—The darker area of the breast, which surrounds the nipple.

Birth control pill—A pill used to ensure that sexual intercourse does not result in pregnancy. Birth control pills are made from artificial estrogens.

Bisexual—A person who engages in sexual activity with members of both sexes.

Boner—A slang expression for an erection.

Castration—Removal of the testes.

Cervix—The narrow opening at the bottom portion of the uterus, which extends into the vagina.

Chancre—A painless, oozing sore, characteristic of the early stages of syphilis.

"Cherry"—Slang term for hymen.

Circumcision—The process in which the foreskin is surgically removed from around the tip of the penis. This is usually done as a way of promoting cleanliness and reducing the risk of infection.

Climax—A commonly used term for orgasm.

Clitoral hood—Tissue from the labia minora that forms a hoodlike covering over the clitoris when a female is sexually aroused.

Clitoris—A small, extremely sensitive female organ located immediately in front of the urethra. Stimulation of the clitoris is often involved in the process of a woman reaching orgasm.

Coitus—A medical term for sexual intercourse.

Coitus interruptus—A very ineffective means of birth control in which the penis is withdrawn from the vagina prior to ejaculation.

Conception—The joining of the male sperm and female ovum to form a fertilized egg.

Condom—Commonly called a rubber or prophylactic. A baglike rubber or membrane covering that is worn on the penis both as a contraceptive device and as a way of protecting against the spread of sexually transmitted diseases.

Contraceptive—Any device used to minimize the possibility of pregnancy as a result of sexual intercourse.

Cross-dresser—Formerly called a transvestite. A person, usually male, who has a strong compulsion to dress in the clothing of the opposite sex.

Cunnilingus—A form of oral sex in which the tongue is used to stimulate the female's vulva.

Diaphragm—A contraceptive device that acts as a cap covering the female's cervix.

Ejaculation—The sudden shooting out of semen from the penis, which almost always occurs when a male experiences orgasm.

Epididymis—A long tube in which the newly developed sperm mature.

Erection—The enlarging and stiffening of the penis as a result of an increased supply of blood to that area. Although erections are usually attributed to sexual stimulation, there are other factors that can cause erections.

Erogenous—Sensitive to sexual excitement. Often used in the term "erogenous zone," which refers to specific areas of the body that are sexually sensitive, such as the lips, breasts, and genitals.

Erotic—Anything that arouses sexual feelings. This term is often used in referring to literature, movies, music, et cetera.

Estrogen—A hormone that produces female sex characteristics. Estrogens also affect the female's menstrual cycle. Birth conrol pills are made from synthetic estrogens.

Fallopian tube—The tubes connecting each ovary with the uterus. Conception usually takes place in this tube.

Fellatio—A form of oral sex in which the mouth makes contact with the male partner's penis.

Female-superior position—A position of sexual intercourse in which the female lies on top of the male.

Fertile—Capable of becoming pregnant.

Fertilization—See Conception.

Fetus—The developing infant inside of the mother, from the eighth week of pregnancy until birth. Before the eighth week it is referred to as an embryo.

Foreplay—The beginning stages of sexual play prior to having sexual intercourse.

Foreskin—The fold of skin that covers the tip of a boy's penis at birth. Often it is removed by circumcision.

Gay—A popularly used term for anything having to do with homosexuals.

Genitals—The external sex organs of both males and females.

Gland—An organ of the body that produces a secretion.

Glans—The head of the penis.

Gonorrhea—A sexually transmitted disease. Common symptoms in a male include a burning sensation when urinating or a milky discharge from the tip of the penis.

Gynecomastia—A temporary enlarging of the breasts in males. This occurs in about 80 percent of teenage boys going through puberty.

Herpes—A sexually transmitted disease, which has become epidemic in proportions. The most common symptom is painful sores, usually on the genitals.

Heterosexual—A person whose sole or primary sexual attraction is to people of the opposite sex.

Homosexual—A person whose sole or primary sexual attraction is to people of the same sex.

Hormones—Chemical messengers produced by the endocrine glands. They regulate many of the body's activities.

Hymen—A membrane that covers the entrance to the vagina.

Hypoallergenic—Any substance that is designed not to elicit allergic reactions.

Impotence—A condition in which a male is unable to attain an erection sufficient to engage in sexual intercourse.

Intrauterine device—Often referred to as an IUD. A contraceptive device made of metal or plastic, which is inserted by a physician into the woman's uterus.

IUD—See intrauterine device.

"Jerk off"—A slang expression meaning to masturbate.

Labia—The "lips" of a female's genital area. There are two sets of lips. The labia majora are the larger, outer lips, and the labia minora are the smaller, inner lips. Both are part of the vulva.

Lateral position—A position of intercourse in which the couple lies in a side-by-side position, facing each other.

Lesbian—A female homosexual.

Male-superior position—A position of sexual intercourse, often referred to as the missionary position. In this position, the male lies on top of the female.

Mammary glands—The milk-producing glands contained in the female breasts.

Masturbation—Self-pleasuring of one's own genitals to produce sexual excitement and often orgasm.

Menopause—The period when a woman ceases to menstruate. This usually will occur between the ages of forty-five and fifty-five.

Menstrual cycle—A woman's fertility cycle. For many women this cycle is twenty-eight to thirty days, but it can vary considerably between women.

Menstruation—A part of the menstrual cycle in which the inner lining of the uterus, along with a small amount of blood, are eliminated through the vagina. Often referred to as a period.

Molestation—To make forced sexual advances on another person.

Mons pubis—The "pubic mound." The soft mound of tissue just above a female's external genitals.

Nipple—The tip of the breast.

Nocturnal emission—Ejaculation of semen that occurs during periods of sleep. Often referred to as wet dream.

Nursing—The feeding of a child at the mother's breast.

Oral contraceptive—See birth control pill.

Oral sex (oral genital sex)—Any sexual activity that involves contact between the mouth and the genitals. See cunnilingus and fellatio.

Orgasm—The peak experience that occurs at the height of sexual excitement. Often referred to as "coming," or climax.

Ovaries—A pair of sex glands in the female that are responsible for the production of the ovum (egg). In addition, they produce female sex hormones. They are located on each side of the upper portion of the uterus.

Ovulation—The process, approximately once each month, of the ovum breaking through the wall of the ovary in order to begin its journey down the fallopian tube.

Penis—The male sexual organ.

Period—See menstruation.

Petting—Touching by a partner of any of the sensitive sexual areas of the body.

Pregnancy—The time between conception and childbirth, when the embryo or fetus is developing in the uterus.

Premature ejaculation—A sexual difficulty in men, in which ejaculation occurs too quickly, thus making sexual satisfaction difficult for one or both partners.

Prostate gland—Surrounds the male urethra, just below the bladder. This gland is responsible for much of the production of the seminal fluid.

Prosthesis (penile)—A permanent implant, surgically placed into the penis of men who are impotent, which then enables them to get an erection.

Prostitute—Any person who participates in sexual activity for money.

Puberty—The period during which a boy or girl becomes capable of reproduction.

Pubic hair—The curly hair that covers the area above the penis in males and vagina in females. Pubic hair is one of the first signs of the onset of adolescence.

Rape—The forcing of a person to engage in sexual activity against his or her will.

Refractory period—A period that occurs after orgasm in most men during which the male is incapable of having another erection or ejaculation. This period may last anywhere from a few minutes to a few days, depending on such factors as age, health, and degree of sexual excitement.

Rhythm method—A method of birth control in which sexual intercourse is timed to coincide with times when it is thought that fertilization of the female's ovum is unlikely. This tends to be an extremely unreliable form of birth control.

Rubber—A slang term for a condom.

Scrotum—The pouch that contains the two testes.

Semen—A thick, sticky, whitish liquid that spurts from the penis during ejaculation. It includes a mixture of sperm and seminal fluid.

Seminal vesicle—Place in a male's body where the sperm mix with the seminal fluid to form the semen. The seminal vesicles are located near the back of the prostate gland.

Sexual intercourse—The placement of the male's penis into the vagina of the female.

Sexually transmitted diseases—Formerly called venereal diseases. Any of a number of diseases that can be transmitted during the close body contact that occurs with sexual activity. See Gonorrhea, Herpes, and Syphilis.

Sixty-nine—Mutual oral-genital sexual activity. This term is so called because the positions of the bodies during this type of sexual activity somewhat resemble the figure 69.

Smegma—A cheeselike substance produced by small glands near the tip of the penis. In uncircumcised males the smegma can accumulate under the foreskin and cause irritation or infection.

Sperm—Microscopic cells that are responsible for fertilizing the female egg (ovum). These reproductive cells are produced by the testes.

Spermicide—A substance used for birth control that, when placed in the female's vagina, kills the sperm before they can meet with the ovum. These substances may be in the form of foams, jellies, creams, or, in a relatively new method, may be placed in a special sponge. Spermicides are often used along with a condom or a diaphragm to ensure that they work more effectively.

Statutory rape—A legal term for sexual intercourse with any child under the age of consent. Often these laws apply only to females under the age of consent. It does not matter whether or not the intercourse was voluntary on the child's part.

STD—A common term used to refer to sexually transmitted diseases.

Sterilization—Any procedure that causes either a male or a female permanently to be unable to produce offspring. Common methods of sterilization are vasectomy in the male and tubal ligation in the female.

Syphilis—A highly contagious sexually transmitted disease. One of the common symptoms during the early stages of this disease are chancres. These disappear as the disease enters the more dangerous later stages.

Testes—Two lumps inside the scrotum, which are often referred to informally as "balls." They are not solid, but rather are made up of spaghettilike tubes.

Testicles—Another name for the testes and scrotum when they are referred to together.

Testosterone—The primary male sex hormone. See Androgen.

Transsexual—A person who biologically is born with one gender (sex), but constantly feels that he or she is trapped in the body of the wrong sex. Surgical procedures to change the sex of the person are often performed.

Transvestite—See Cross-dresser.

Tubal ligation—The most common method of surgical sterilization performed on females. In this method, the fallopian tubes are cut so the ova cannot meet with the sperm.

Urethra—The tube through which urine is discharged from the body. In the male it is also used to ejaculate the semen.

Uterus—The womb. The organ that holds the growing baby during pregnancy.

Vagina—The tube that connects the uterus with the vulva. During sexual intercourse, the erect penis is placed into the vagina. During childbirth, the vagina acts as the birth canal through which the newborn child is delivered.

Vas deferens—The sperm duct. After the sperm are produced, the stronger sperm are moved by microscopic hairs through this sperm duct until they mix with the rest of the sticky liquid that makes up the semen.

Vasectomy—The cutting of the vas deferens. This is done on men as a form of birth control. After a vasectomy a male still ejaculates the seminal fluid, but without the sperm, which are responsible for reproduction.

Venereal diseases—See Sexually transmitted diseases.

Virgin—A person, male or female, who previously has not engaged in sexual intercourse.

Vulva—The woman's external sex organs. This includes the labia majora, labia minora, clitoris, and the opening to the vagina.

Wet dream—See nocturnal emission.

NOTES

1. Bill Cosby, "The Regular Way," *Playboy*, December 1968, pp. 288–89.
2. Aaron Hass, Ph.D., *Teenage Sexuality* (New York: Pinnacle Books, 1981), p. 210.
3. Shere Hite, *The Hite Report on Male Sexuality* (New York: Alfred A. Knopf, 1981), p. 395.
4. Julius Lester, "Being A Boy," *Ms.*, July 1973, p. 113.
5. Bernie Zilbergeld, Ph.D., *Male Sexuality* (Boston: Little, Brown, 1978), p. 135.
6. Shere Hite, p. 485.
7. A. C. Kinsey, W. B. Pomeroy, and C. E. Martin, *Sexual Behavior in the Human Male* (Philadelphia: W.B. Saunders, 1948), p. 502.
8. Shere Hite, p. 487.
9. Aaron Hass, p. 57.
10. Cameron Crowe, *Fast Times at Ridgemont High: A True Story* (New York: Simon and Schuster, 1981), pp. 160–62.
11. Herant A. Katchadourian and Donald T. Lunde, *Fundamentals of Human Sexuality* (New York: Holt, Rinehart and Winston, 1972), pp. 427, 439.
12. Timothy W. Gallwey, *The Inner Game of Tennis* (New York: Random House, 1974), p. 51.

INDEX

NOTE: *Page numbers in italics indicate illustrations.*

To the reader:

If you have any questions about the information covered in this book or would like to offer your opinion of how you liked it, please write to the author at the following address:

Jay Gale, Ph.D.
P.O. Box 3673
Mission Viejo, CA 92690